BETWEEN HOME AND NURSING HOME

Golden Age Books
Perspective on Aging
Series Editor: Steven L. Mitchell

After the Stroke: Coping with America's Third Leading Cause of Death
by Evelyn Shirk

The Age of Aging: A Reader in Social Gerontology
edited by Abraham Monk

Caring for an Aging Parent: Have I Done All I Can?
by Avis Jane Ball

Caring for the Alzheimer Patient: A Practical Guide (Second Edition)
edited by Raye Lynn Dippel, Ph.D.
and J. Thomas Hutton, M.D., Ph.D.

Caring for the Parkinson Patient: A Practical Guide
by J. Thomas Hutton, M.D., Ph.D.
and Raye Lynne Dippel, Ph.D.

Eldercare: Coping with Late-Life Crisis
by James Kenny, Ph.D., and Stephen Spicer, M.D.

Handle With Care: A Question of Alzheimer's
by Dorothy S. Brown

My Parents Never Had Sex: Myths and Facts of Sexual Aging
by Doris B. Hammond, Ph.D.

On Our Own: Independent Living for Older Persons
by Ursula A. Falk, Ph.D.

Promises to Keep: The Family's Role in Nursing Home Care
by Katherine L. Karr

Understanding "Senility": A Layperson's Guide
by Virginia Fraser and Susan M. Thornton

When Blind Eyes Pierce the Darkness: A Mother's Insights
Compiled by Peter A. Angeles

Working with the Elderly: An Introduction
edited by Elizabeth S. Deichman, Ed.M., OTR
and Regina Kociecki, B.S.

You, Your Parent and the Nursing Home
by Nancy Fox

BETWEEN HOME AND NURSING HOME

THE BOARD AND CARE ALTERNATIVE

Ivy M. Down, M.A., and
Lorraine Schnurr, Ph.D.

PROMETHEUS BOOKS
Buffalo • New York

Published 1991 by Prometheus Books

95 94 93 92 91   5 4 3 2 1

Library of Congress Cataloging-in-Publication Data

Down, Ivy.
    Between home and nursing home : the board and care-alternative /
by Ivy Down and Lorraine Schnurr.
        p.   cm. — (Golden age books)
    Includes bibliographical references.
    ISBN 0-87975-619-5 (cloth : acid free)
    ISBN 0-87975-620-9 (paper : acid free)
    1. Old age homes—United States—Activity programs. 2. Social work with
the aged—United States. 3. Aged—Care—United States. I. Schnurr, Lorraine.
II. Title. III. Series.
HV1454.2.U6D68   1991
362.6′3—dc20   91-21157
                                                                      CIP

Printed on acid-free paper in the United States of America

Foreword

Residential care facilities, or "board and care homes," have been a refuge for the elderly, the disabled, and the mentally ill for a long time. The quality of care provided by some of these homes has been dismal and disgraceful in the past. Nevertheless, they constitute a viable and necessary housing alternative. Once residents are housed, however, little mental stimulation is provided to them, which leads to further mental deterioration and physical atrophy.

Between Home and Nursing Home contains exercises and activities designed to stimulate the senses of touch, taste, hearing, sight, and smell in an easy, straightforward format. This book will do more than assist board and care owners/operators and caregivers to provide stimulating activities for residents; it will raise public awareness about what *should be done* and what *needs to be done* in board and cares. Those who advocate for the elderly will find much here to address for a long time to come, and individuals seeking board and care placement for a friend or a relative will discover valuable ideas on how to proceed. This book is a reference and a resource, a welcome addition to the literature covering a much-neglected subject.

Jack York, M.D., Psychiatrist
Mental Health Administrator
Highland General Hospital
Oakland, California

Contents

Foreword *by Jack York, M.D.*   5

Acknowledgments   9

Introduction   11

1. What Are Board and Care Facilities?   21

2. Case Management   45

3. Sensory Deprivation and Its Consequences   59

4. Memory Loss and Mental Health   93

5. Spiritual Health   111

6. Art Therapy   119

7. Music Therapy   142

8. Physical Exercise   149

9. Miscellaneous Activities   166

10. Some Final Thoughts   177

8   Contents

Appendix 1: What You Need to Know about Retirement Facilities   181

Appendix 2: A Checklist to Take with You
When You Visit a Residential Care Facility   184

Appendix 3: State Units on Aging   187

Appendix 4: State Agencies with Jurisdiction over
Residential Care Facilities   193

Appendix 5: State Long-Term Care Ombudsman   201

Appendix 6: A Sample Order of Worship   208

Appendix 7: Songs for Music Therapy   210

Appendix 8: Friendly Visitors   215

Acknowledgments

We are grateful to the many authors and publishers whose materials are quoted, cited, referenced, or recommended in this volume, and to those manufacturers whose products are discussed. A special debt is owed to those whose work in the area of sensory deprivation and stimulation has shed much-needed light in this new and as yet underdeveloped area of research.

We thank Carmel Sheridan and Elenore Ashworth for sharing their carefully thought out exercises to help elders remain alert. Mental and emotional fitness is just as important as physical well-being. Both authors offer step-by-step instructions that are easy for staff and residents to follow. In his book *Human Options,* Norman Cousins says: "Laughter is a form of internal jogging."[1] If we stop to analyze what happens to our bodies when something strikes us as funny and we burst out in a hearty belly-laugh, the analogy Mr. Cousins offers can be readily appreciated. The staff of the Ethel Percy Andrus Gerontology Center at the University of Southern California (Los Angeles) developed and published *Humor: The Tonic You Can Afford,* which shows how to use humor to make life more enjoyable. We are indebted to them for their permission to reference portions of it in our discussion. The humor hour that we recommend for every board and care can be a daily event of inestimable value yet costs very little in terms of money and effort. It's also just plain fun!

The creative imagery of *Hanimals,* by Roberto Marchiori and Mario Mariotti, is a fun activity that can be led by any board and care staff member. We thank Green Tiger Press and the creators of Hanimals for permission to share their work with our readers. Hanimals can be the basis for both active physical involvement and mentally stimulating exercise.

9

When the KOOSH Ball® came on the market, we found it to be useful as a hand exerciser and just a fun object to watch (eye exerciser). Its "giggle factor" among residents was so high that we asked its creators if we might share the fun with our readers. We thank the manufacturers for their permission.

Although some of the books we suggest in the annotated resource bibliographies at the end of each chapter may not be available in your local library, others that closely approximate them in content most probably are. Your librarian or local bookstore manager should be able to help you locate pertinent materials. For those chapters in which a variety of topics are covered we list the resources according to the section for which they are most pertinent: e.g., materials to assist the hearing impaired, resources to stimulate memory and mental activity, arts and crafts materials.

We also wish to thank cartoonist Sarley and the Hearing Society for the Bay Area, Inc., for permission to use their "Tips for Talking to the Hard of Hearing" and other suggestions for easier ways to communicate with those who are hearing impaired. Sarley's cartoons remind us of the many thoughtless things we do when interacting with someone who has a hearing deficit. Maybe his humorous efforts will help all of us change our habits.

Finally, our thanks go to Ms. Eleanor Hull, Project Coordinator with the City of Oakland's Office of Aging, for her support of our project.

Our friend Nelson Keeler, retired from the Surgeon General's office, spent many hours reading the manuscript of this book and suggested ways to make it easier to follow. We thank him for his interest and help. It is with gratitude that we acknowledge our many friends and associates in the gerontology field who offered their encouragement.

The editors of Prometheus Books suggested that we expand our original focus and by doing so we have increased the value of the project. We are especially grateful to our editor, Steven L. Mitchell, for his comments and suggestions.

NOTE

1. Norman Cousins, *Human Options* (New York: Berkeley Books, 1981), p. 217.

Introduction

This book took shape as we shared with one another our professional experiences accumulated over many years of working with board and care residents and our contact with operators, owners, and managers. Focusing on the apathy and deterioration of residents, we came to the conclusion that our training and hands-on experience in the field have given us the background and understanding needed to address the proper functions of board and care facilities, to evaluate their usefulness as a housing alternative for the nation's elderly, and to highlight some of the problems they face.

In presenting this volume, our intention is to offer encouragement and helpful advice to elders who currently live in board and care homes, to the families of these residents as well as prospective new clients, to the people who operate or manage such facilities, and to the professionals whose job it is to locate appropriate living arrangements for the increasing numbers of elderly or disabled individuals who can no longer live alone in safety.

Who is in need of this kind of living arrangement? As we shall see, generally speaking, board and care residents consist of persons who are basically able to care for themselves but could use some help with such daily activities as grooming, bathing, or personal care. Others may require help managing medications, obtaining personal care items, handling daily finances, and related activities that fall under the category of "instrumental activities" of daily living. For the most part, however, the vast majority of these elders are quite capable of doing a great many things for themselves and do not need the full-time, skilled health-care services of a nursing home or a convalescent hospital.

In addition, our purpose is to offer helpful resource materials that might be called upon for assistance in seeing to the needs of those who require this intermediate level of care. These sources will not constitute a definitive listing by any stretch of the imagination, but they should suggest possibilities that readers can pursue in their own states, counties, cities, and towns. For those individuals who plan activities or are in a position to encourage managers of facilities to do so, we hope that these suggested resources prove useful. We offer them while remaining mindful of residents' broad range of abilities and the spectrum of capacities demonstrated by the operators of residential care facilities, their staffs, and the volunteers or family members who may provide assistance.

Furthermore, we offer operators of board snd cares help with licensing requirements pertaining to activities for residents. Since we are most familiar with the regulations of our home state of California (which has more than six thousand board and care facilities operating within its jurisdiction), the discussion of needs and services is in accordance with the regulations of the California State Adult Residential Care facilities licensing requirements[1] Section 85079, which state:

> The Licensee [the board and care or residential care facility operator] shall insure that planned recreational activities which include the following are provided for their clients:
>
> (1) Activities that require group interaction;
> (2) Physical activities—including but not limited to games, sports and exercises;
> (3) In facilities with a licensed capacity of 50 or more clients, a current, written program of activities shall be planned in advance and made available to all clients;
> (4) Activities shall be encouraged through provision of the space, equipment, and supplies specified in Section 85087.2, 85087.3 and 85087.9 (g).

Assuming your state has a statute that makes provision for the licensing of board and care facilities under its jurisdiction,* the wording of the requirements are likely to differ somewhat. However, if your state does not have regulations similar to the above, advocacy groups for the elderly, as well as other interested parties, should lobby their state legislatures for

---

*The agencies listed in Appendix 4 should be of some help in determining the applicable law in your state.

clearly defined legal requirements. Having statewide licensing requirements can help guarantee that more board and cares will be held to a minimum standard of policies, practices, procedures, and services.

When this book was originally conceived we focused on persons now living in board and cares who, although recipients of basic care to help with the activities of daily living, had little or no opportunity for activities that would stimulate the five senses—sight, hearing, taste, smell, and touch—the essential faculties that help all of us function effectively from day to day. We wanted to show that, beyond the requirements of basic care, there are ways for people to retain a wide array of capacities in spite of their many and varied disabilities, as long as their sensory faculties continue to be exercised on a regular basis. We intended to offer activities through art and music as well as mental, physical, and spiritual exercises that would stimulate the senses and keep even those with limited abilities functioning well. After all, our senses, much like our muscles and our minds, must be exercised regularly if they are to serve us.

As we looked into the essential components of board and cares, we realized that there are many areas in which readers need help. Not only could such a volume assist present and future proprietors of board and care homes, but also families who are faced with the frustrating task of finding a safe place for an aging parent or relative. We could help social workers and case managers who must relocate elderly or disabled clients whose physical and/or mental limitations make it unsafe for them to continue living at home alone. Those who serve in hospital discharge programs may also find a discussion of board and cares useful when in need of finding alternative care arrangements for elderly patients who would not be able to care for themselves adequately if returned to their homes, yet do not require the extensive full-time skilled care that nursing homes provide. Concerned members of the community who want to help ensure a good quality of life for those who can no longer fully care for themselves will find our discussion of board and cares useful in their efforts to make a more knowledgeable choice about alternative care facilities. They will become familiar with the kinds of care currently offered and what to expect when a board and care is chosen. The extensive Appendices contain, among other things, a detailed list of what to look for in a residential care facility and a short checklist to accompany those who are evaluating a prospective home.

WHO NEEDS BOARD AND CARES?

When faced with the prospect of leaving home or an apartment to seek out alternative living and/or care arrangements, the more affluent elderly have a number of options open to them. They can buy into a multi-service retirement community whose amenities range from total independent living, through various levels of intermediate care, to full-time, skilled nursing care when it is needed. Alternatively, older adults with ample resources can hire a private-duty health-care aide or a certified nursing assistant. If need be, they can even relocate to areas where the services they seek are more readily available.

For the vast majority of elders living in the United States—most of whom are female and former homemakers with little if any income beyond that which they receive from Social Security—board and cares offer one of the few viable, cost-effective alternatives to both nursing home placement and costly in-home care. This volume offers older persons and those who provide support and varying levels of care (e.g., the family, church, doctor, social worker, etc.) the kind of information they will need to help them plan for and select a suitable licensed and supervised facility. In the pages that follow, we suggest what to look for in a facility, what kinds of services are (or should be) provided, and what level of supervision to expect so that our oldest citizens can have the best chance of enjoying a good quality of life in spite of their disabilities.

Quality of life is a subjective concept, often hard to define, yet much desired and sought after. Most of us do have a sense of what it means, though we may disagree about specific elements of the definition. However we come to define the concept for ourselves, quality of life has a universal component: no matter what the nature or extent of a person's disabilities, that individual deserves the oppoi unity to get as much out of life as possible, regardless of the obstacles to be faced. Those in the helping professions should have as their first priority the goal of securing the best quality of life possible for each client. As coauthors of this book, it is our firm belief that a good "quality of life" for the elderly has been neglected by many who provide services to our aging population. To remedy this deficit, we address the matter directly and constructively. We believe—no, we *know*—that a good quality of life for America's elderly is possible in today's board and care homes.

SOME QUESTIONS

Caregiving for the elderly has become a growth industry: with ever-increasing numbers of older persons and family caregivers confronting difficult choices about types of living arrangements and levels of care for those who are experiencing diminished or reduced capacity, various housing and eldercare alternatives have been devised. Amid the plethora of prospects, from skilled care to in-home service providers, stands the board and care home.

But how do these board and cares differ from nursing homes? Why would board and cares be a more suitable type of living arrangement for many of our nation's older adults? For whom would these homes be a good alternative care option? What services, if any, *must* these facilities offer? What services *should* they provide? What can board and care owners, operators, and/or managers do to maximize the physical and mental well-being of their residents? Realistically, what sorts of care options, services, and activities could board and care managers structure into the daily routine of the residents? What kinds of activities would help elders who live in such facilities to continue to maintain, if not expand or enhance, the use of their mental, physical, and emotional capacities? What would encourage residents to use their sensory faculties and thereby increase individual levels of functioning and alertness? What would help to prevent many of our nation's elderly from rapidly declining to that state of apathy, despair, and depression which so quickly envelops people when they lose control over their lives? How can elderly board and care residents achieve the highest levels of personal control even when mobility becomes limited, restricted, or (in some cases) severely reduced? How can older persons realistically expect to remain alert to and involved in the world around them when so much of what they had once considered "normal" appears beyond their grasp?

These are some of the questions we will focus upon throughout this book. While our answers ought not to be construed as definitive, we do believe that sharing the insights we have gained from years of experience with board and care facilities and their residents may heighten the awareness of the elderly, family members, caregivers (whether professional, familial, or volunteer), and prospective board and care operators to the methods, practices, and services that have worked to help a great many older adults live the fullest life possible.

Ivy Down's interest in this project grew out of her efforts, both as a staff person and as a volunteer, to develop community services that could improve the lives of elders. Before settling in the San Francisco

Bay Area, she had seen elders in a variety of situations, many of whom she felt were capable of performing the activities of daily living for themselves. These persons were oftentimes confined to nursing homes because their families had no idea where to find or how to obtain help for their relatives who were in need of care and supervision. For some people, there were few, if any, options when advanced age and diminished capacity made living alone virtually impossible. The board and care alternative was not open to them.

Furthermore, Ivy had been exposed to both health-preserving and health-destroying facilities: the real difference between them often resting upon the operators' willingness not only to recognize residents' needs for stimulating activities but actually to make an effort toward providing them. Less willing proprietors/managers/operators feel that the commitment to provide basic care fulfills their primary responsibilities to families and residents alike. This book will help the owners/managers of smaller board and cares to lead activities even though they cannot afford to hire trained activities directors, and are themselves neither skilled nor trained in this area.

Lorraine Schnurr is in daily contact with Licensed Vocational Nurses, Certified Nurses Assistants, and nurse's aides who care for disabled elders. Feedback from these professionals testifies to the presence of an urgent need for developing ways to stop the continued decline in physical, mental, and emotional well-being among resident populations of community-based adult care facilities. A deep concern for the deterioration of our nation's elderly led her to look for ways to help put an end to this progressive decline.

Lorraine recalls a very attractive and independent aunt who, as her own family drifted away, invited into her home an elderly friend who needed a place to stay because he wasn't able to take care of himself quite as well as he would have liked. As word spread of her neighborliness, others asked if they might rent a room. What a wonderful friend she was, and how helpful she could be.

Actually, this is how many board and cares started: After many years of living with a spouse and/or family, someone—usually a woman between the ages of forty and sixty—with a large house, whose family had moved away, made the conscious choice to share empty or spare rooms with elderly friends in need of safe, affordable housing. The owner/landlord provides basic needs such as meals and maybe some assistance with personal care, but may also choose to offer a range of services—for example, basic cleaning, laundry, and possibly even occasional transportation to health and beauty appointments or to shopping areas. The room provided and the services offered could be exchanged for companionship, for help around the house, or for an agreed upon amount of rent. Then, as other older persons seek out living arrangements and services of a similar nature, the owner might expand to accommodate more tenants, eventually becoming a licensed operator of a board and care (though the residence may not officially refer to itself by this name).

Since your coauthors have worked to develop services for elders in the San Francisco Bay Area and each of us has experience in the growth of organizations to meet the needs of this increasing population, we have been able to monitor the trends. We have taken note of the increased longevity older people are experiencing year after year. In the "Newsbriefs" section of *Aging Connection,* a publication produced by the American Society on Aging, the editors focus on this important point:

> More older people will live alone in the twenty-first century, says a new forecast from the Urban Institute. Expect 20 million solo elders in America in 2030, compared with 8.4 million in 1984. Fewer marriages, fewer children and more divorces will force up the number, says the report. If the current disability rate persists, those needing institutional care will more than triple from 1.3 million in 1984 to 5.3 million in 2030.[2]

Furthermore, an *Older Americans Report,* a survey by the U.S. Senate Special Committee on Aging, shows medical costs nationwide to be

> the highest among the major industries, (and) cut into pensions severely. In addition, 31 percent of all elders depend on Social Security for at least 80 percent of their income, and older persons are more likely than the nonelderly to live just above the poverty line.[3]

The implication of this research reinforces our finding that moderate- and low-income elders will be even more in need of the kind of housing that board and care homes are able to provide. With this in mind, we have carefully studied the board and care concept and have formulated some basic guidelines concerning what the components of their design should be, including services, activities, and the importance of establishing a health-enhancing environment.

Individuals who are considering alternative living and/or care arrangements can use the present volume as a handy guide showing them what to look for and, with its help, be in a better position to ask intelligent questions when evaluating a board and care or related residential facility. It is our hope that a discussion of this innovative housing and care option will prod people to consider it carefully and to plan ahead. Preparing for the future is particularly important for older adult children whose parents are reaching advanced age. When considered judgment rather than chance, panic, or desperation inform our choices, both the decision-making process and the eventual selection of an appropriate facility are arrived at comfortably and with a welcome sense of assurance that accompanies thoughtful deliberation.

Ms. Ruby MacDonald, a writer and the owner of Chateau Pleasant Hills, a retirement complex in California, developed a brief list of suggestions to help those who are seriously considering making a choice from among the many available housing and care options. With her kind permission we have included it as our Appendix 1.[4] Whether you are seeking new living arrangements for yourself, a spouse, a parent, or a friend, there is much insight to be gained by reading and following her suggestions carefully.

In her publication titled "When Care Is Needed," Dorothy Epstein provides the California Ombudsman program with "A checklist to Take with You When You Visit a Residential Care Facility."[5] With her permission, we have included it as our Appendix 2 in the hope that it will provide added assistance to those who will be investigating various facilities. Although every item on her list may not apply directly to the board and care homes in your area, most of the checklist is pertinent and will help inform prospective residents about aspects of facilities that would otherwise remain overlooked. We hope that the questions Ms. Epstein poses will help readers make the choice best suited to their needs and those of their loved ones.

Many older persons, as well as concerned caregivers and health-care specialists, eventually realize that they must have help to address their own housing and care needs or those of a loved one or client. They want to locate a safer living environment that will fit their desire for independence while at the same time meet their particular needs for appropriate levels of care. Families who seek the best care for their aging relatives can, with some help, locate a facility that will approach or achieve the type of care they desire, at a price the elder can afford. This facility should be located in an area that is convenient for family members to keep close watch and feel secure that their loved one is well cared for.

The board and care phenomenon has resulted in a fast-growing industry. For that reason new laws are being developed and introduced in many states to ensure that these homes for the elderly meet specific health and safety standards. Changes in the residential care field take place as advocacy groups raise the community's awareness about what needs to be done to improve services and physical facilities. You, too, can help by becoming knowledgeable about conditions in board and care homes in your area. It is our fervent hope that this volume will encourage more people to recognize the potential health care and housing benefits of board and care facilities. We further hope that it will encourage communities across the nation to help board and cares live up to their potential as alternative housing and care providers for our aging population.

NOTES

1. Licensing Requirements: "Operating Without a License," State of California Regulations on Community Care Licensure Requirements, *CARCH News* (March 1988):17-19.

2. The American Society on Aging, "Newsbriefs," in *The Aging Connection* (February/March 1990).

3. Ibid.

4. Ruby MacDonald, "What You Need to Know about Retirement Facilities," *Senior Spectrum* (August 1988).

5. Dorothy Epstein, "A Checklist to Take with You When You Visit a Residential Care Facility," published by Ombudsman, Inc., of Alameda County with support from the State Ombudsman Program and the Department of Aging.

1

What Are Board and Care Facilities?

Though they have existed in various forms for decades, there is still some misunderstanding today over the nature and intended purpose of the residential care facilities for the elderly (RCFEs) known as "board and cares." There are several reasons for this confusion. The term suggests that they are modern adaptations of the familiar types of boarding or rooming houses where, for the price of weekly or monthly rent, guests were provided sparsely furnished but adequate rooms, along with meals, bathroom facilities, and possibly some light cleaning. But we are not concerned here with mere accommodations for the night or even for a few weeks; and the clientele does not consist of traveling salesmen, transient workers, or out-of-town guests. Board and cares constitute a community-based residential living and caregiving arrangement that has developed to help serve the complex needs of America's rapidly increasing elderly population.

The board and care option serves as a cost-effective alternative for many older adults who live alone on a fixed income and find it increasingly difficult to take care of their homes/apartments and their own personal daily needs. Some of these elders may have outlived their families and most of their friends: they are isolated, alone, and in need of basic companionship. Those who do have families often prefer not to impose on their loved ones: instead, they seek to remain independent for as long as possible until physical decline and diminished capacity make it necessary to enter a nursing home. Board and care homes are one of the few accessible alternative living arrangements available to the elderly and to concerned family members who recognize the need to locate accommodations that provide essential services and appropriate levels of care but do not consider their care needs to be so significant as to warrant the more serious and costly step of nursing home placement.

In those states and localities where they exist, pertinent laws and ordinances governing community-based residential care facilities refer to board and cares by any number of names and incorporate a variety of criteria when defining such facilities. We define a board and care home as: *a place to live where elder residents are provided sleeping accommodations, meals, some help with activities of daily living (such as bathing and grooming) and with instrumental activities (such as assistance with transportation and medication).* According to a 1988 publication entitled *A Home Away From Home,* produced by the American Association of Retired Persons (AARP), board and care facilities provide "a living arrangement in which a resident is provided room, meals, help with activities of daily living, and some protective supervision."[1]

Board and cares operate under a variety of names depending upon the state in which they are located; the more common names include: adult foster homes, group homes, homes for the aged, rest homes, care or personal care homes, or domiciliaries. In California, the State Department of Social Services' Community Care Licensing Division Information System (CCLDIS) has lists of all *licensed* "Community Care Facilities." Although the names under which these facilities operate may vary dramatically, the concept of a board and care is still applicable, provided that the residence conforms to the basic working definition set forth above.

In California, the CCLDIS lists are printed for each county; every city in a given county has listed under its name some vital information on all care facilities: the administrator's name and the licensee's name, along with a brief description of services provided, specific requirements for admission (e.g., age and physical condition), and the facility's maximum resident capacity. Using the city of Oakland as an example, a quick look at the list for Alameda County provides a roster of facilities in the Oakland area. Assuming that one needed to find a community-based board and care for an elderly aunt, one could look under "Facility Type: Residential—Elderly" and peruse three pages of listed facilities, complete with addresses and telephone numbers. One home shows the age range of clients to be sixty-two years or older; the number of ambulatory (those able to walk unassisted); semi-ambulatory (those who need assistance moving about); and nonambulatory (confined to bed) residents; and the home's total capacity. With this information in hand, interested persons are then able to call and make an appointment to visit the facility, knowing beforehand the major requirements for admission and a few specifics about the resident population.

A similar list of residential care facilities is available from any state's Department of Social Services, Department of Aging, or Community Care Licensing Division (see Appendices 3, 4, and 5 for appropriate contacts in your state). If all relevant information is available, any prospective resident, or interested family member seeking to place a relative, should be able to contact the home(s) in their immediate vicinity. Your community's Social Services Agency may be the quickest route to this information; in rural areas, the County Social Services Agency should be contacted to secure a list of local facilities. If you are unable to locate this information, contact your state's Department of Social Services. In the event that your state has not developed such a list, perhaps you can join with others who are similarly concerned and voice the need to have such information readily available. As America's elderly population increases each year, more and more pressure will be brought to bear upon state agencies to compile lists of board and care facilities for individuals and community service providers so that the housing and care needs of our older citizens can be adequately met.

The State of California lists all *licensed* residential care facilities; state law requires that all board and cares with six or more residents be licensed. As carefully drafted as this legislation is, there are many small homes that escape even the minimal supervision that licensing regulations can provide. Traditional board and cares, then, may range in size and capacity from a small private home accommodating just three or four elders to larger, formerly single-family dwellings that can serve the needs of six or more elders. In recent years, however, the concept of residential care has been extended to include large facilities, planned and built for congregate living, many of which contain fifty to one hundred or more residents.

A licensed board and care will be supervised by the state's Board of Health or possibly the Social Services Department, and may also be monitored by an ombudsman.* This does not necessarily mean that because

---

*Each state has a Long-Term Care Ombudsman Program with a local ombudsman assigned to designated regions of the state. An ombudsman acts as a liaison between the state, the licensed (and unlicensed) facilities, and the community. Individuals who serve in this capacity attempt to address concerns and complaints raised by residents as well as operators/managers, families, and the community at large. This is often accomplished by investigating the matter and having it addressed by the facility. When this fails, or is not an appropriate course of action, then the ombudsman contacts the agencies (local, state, or federal) best able to focus on and remedy the particular problem or need.

a small facility is not licensed, it is substandard, unsafe, or otherwise unsatisfactory. Because unlicensed facilities (those with numbers of residents below a state's mandated minimum) may not be supervised, they can be—and many often are—in violation of health, fire, or building codes. On the other hand, these homes may simply be too small and are thus overlooked by regulatory agencies whose jurisdiction does not extend to them. This is not to suggest that all small board and cares are inadequate or unsafe; in fact, they may be just what many families need. So don't overlook them in your search for the best housing and care arrangement for an elderly relative.* Many prospective residents and their families or caregivers feel more secure about community-based residences if these facilities are accountable to government agencies that inspect and monitor staff, services, and levels of care.

The list of community care facilities for Alameda County shows that in 1989 there were 193 licensed residential facilities for elderly persons, six of which were large homes with between 125 and 300 residents. Such homes have a wide range of staff to assist their clients, including an activities director, registered nurses (possibly licensed practical nurses as well) and aides, housekeeping and maintenance workers, kitchen and dining room help, and administrative personnel. On the other end of the spectrum, one finds the smaller board and cares—by far the largest segment of the industry—which generally accommodate from six to ten elders. Here the staff may consist of an all-purpose aide and a cook. These small community-based facilities must rely heavily upon volunteers and community resources if residents are to be given more than basic care. High school and college students/teachers, church groups, and retirees are among the volunteers at these board and cares.

THE COST OF BOARD AND CARE SERVICES

The fees charged to those who live in board and care residential facilities cover a wide range from the modestly priced homes that offer little more than a place to stay and meals, to more moderately priced residences that add a few basic services such as cleaning and laundry, to more expensive

---

*If the state where you reside lists only licensed facilities, you may have to search a bit to find the smaller residential care providers in your area. Since they are in contact with many facilities, licensed and unlicensed, your long-term care ombudsman should probably be the focus of your inquiry.

facilities that offer a wide array of amenities. Actual monthly rates vary depending upon the specific characteristics and features of the facility: location, desirability, quality of accommodations and services provided. Like all landlord-tenant agreements, the rate to be paid is set by the owner/operator: monthly fees range across a wide spectrum—from several hundred dollars to well over a thousand. The figure actually paid will depend on whether all available services are included in the rental fee or if some are optional and can be added at the resident's request. Naturally, the latter will increase the cost of an elder's stay. Not surprisingly, the more expensive homes attract only the more affluent older adults.

In living arrangements known as "retirement complexes," the monthly charges range from $1,000 to $1,500. They cover many of the same specific services offered by more expensive housing options—for example, meals, laundry, cleaning, health care access, socialization activities, and transportation services. Some of these congregate living arrangements provide clients with the opportunity to move up to a higher level of care, including part- or full-time skilled nursing, as the need arises and health-care requirements demand.

For the vast majority of elders, however, the more costly alternative living arrangements are not viable options. Most older people need housing and assistive services that can be obtained at a much lower cost. As the report of the Senate Special Committee on Aging shows, 31 percent of all elders depend on Social Security for at least 80 percent of their income.[2] By far the largest percentage of America's current elderly population consists of female former homemakers, the vast majority of whom, throughout their preretirement years, engaged in little if any outside employment that could have provided them with a separate pension of their own. These persons cannot afford higher-priced private retirement homes or apartment complexes, and little if any federally subsidized housing is available through the Department of Housing and Urban Development (HUD).* Where such housing does exist, it is in great demand, with long waiting lists. In addition, those elders with modest means are unable to rely on health insurance plans to assist in paying for their board and care stay: unlike nursing homes, board and cares, though often considerably less expensive and more appropriate for the specific individual needs of many elders, are not considered medical facilities and thus are not covered

---

*This federal housing is attractive and desired because those elders who are lucky enough to find it in their area and have their applications accepted only contribute about 30 percent of their income for rent. This permits a modest standard of living to be maintained.

by private forms of third-party reimbursement.[3] Some low-income elderly qualify under Social Security regulations for Supplemental Social Security Income (SSI), which some states augment with additional support to qualified individuals.* But even with this financial assistance, it can be a considerable struggle to find a facility that offers adequate basic accommodations and essential services.

WHO OWNS BOARD AND CARES?

The board and care concept has its roots in history: at various times financial need has forced many people in late middle age to make use of empty bedrooms in their homes. As we can see, the board and care (or residential care) option does appear to be a clear extension of the boarding house phenomenon. Older couples or widowed females found themselves inhabiting large houses with many empty rooms once occupied by children who had long since left home to find their own way in life. The need for additional income, along with a desire for companionship, made the idea of renting out rooms a sensible alternative to giving up a home in which so much had been invested. The homeowner would then agree to take in parents, other relatives, or elderly friends. As people in the surrounding area eventually found themselves in need of a homelike atmosphere for their aging relatives, inquiries might be made to determine if the homeowner had additional space available. The capacity of such homes depended on the number of rooms for rent and the number of elderly residents the owner felt he or she could be adequately accommodate.

While the community-based residential care phenomenon has enjoyed a solid grassroots tradition, the high cost of real estate in many areas make it increasingly difficult for someone to buy a large, older home for the purpose of starting a board and care. The cost of renovations needed to bring a structure up to state health, fire, safety, and community care facility standards is considerable, and for some people prohibitive. With starting costs of this magnitude, the monthly fee for residents would necessarily be quite high.

A number of large residential care facilities have been started by church or civic organizations (e.g., the Masons and the Lions clubs). The Salem Lutheran Home in Oakland, California, began when the staffs of two

---

*Whether or not an elder can even get aid and, if so, the amount to which the person is eligible depends upon the state of residence.

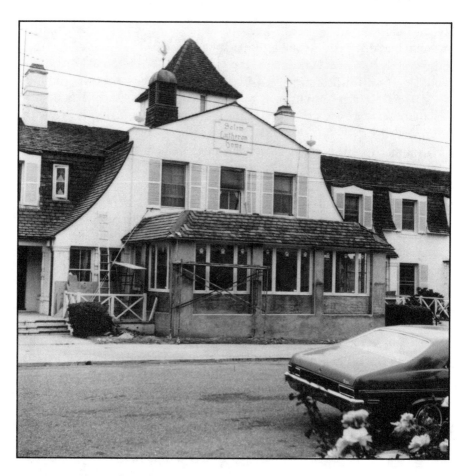

large Lutheran churches realized that there was a need to accommodate those of their members who could no longer live comfortably or safely on their own. The churches organized and planned, bought land and existing homes, and eventually became part of a larger group of Lutheran retirement complexes now called California Lutheran Homes. Over the years, Salem Home was renovated as needed and new buildings were constructed, creating a warm, friendly, and safe living environment for elders.

In Oakland, just across the Bay from San Francisco, Methodists, Baptists, Episcopalians, and many other denominations have built retirement facilities at which residents pay moderate to high monthly rates. Some labor unions also have their own retirement homes. And the HUD-subsidized residences for low-income elders—in Oakland they are called Satellite

Homes—number seven in all. Each of these facilities is large enough to hire activities directors as well as other support staff.

Some board and care homes are "for-profit" while others are "non-profit" or "not-for-profit." It is best to inquire with your own community's Social Service Department to find out the kinds of residential care facilities near you. (A list of the state agencies for the aging is provided in Appendix 3.)

Another more recent development in retirement housing is the blossoming of large complexes built specifically for this purpose. Land is purchased, buildings erected, and the facility is marketed to interested purchasers. These are "for-profit" businesses; there are even chains of them with the same corporation building large-capacity structures in different locations—a growing health-care phenomenon. After evaluating population statistics and demographic predictions, corporations have anticipated a need and sought to provide facilities to meet it. The target market here is the more affluent retired person; developers have anticipated the types of amenities that these potential residents may require or demand and have built them into the construction plans from the beginning. For those older adults who can afford the high cost, such congregate housing units are admittedly wonderful developments. However, these retirement havens become safe and comfortable islands, often divorced from the traditional multiracial, multigenerational communities from which so many elderly have come. Future problems may surface when different age groups— and often racial or ethnic groups—begin living apart from the broader community. However, for a growing number of elders, many of whom realize their own increased vulnerability, these multiunit housing complexes offer an appealing sense of security.

Another type of board and care developer is the community organization that serves the elderly. Such groups may buy a large existing home and remodel it specifically for the purpose of providing housing for various frail elders who do not need full-time skilled nursing care. The board and care homes of these groups usually have a common purpose: for example, focusing on older residents who share the same language or culture. In one case, a Japanese-American senior services organization bought a large older home that could accommodate from six to ten elders. The seller, who had an aged mother, was sympathetic to the needs of others similarly situated. He willingly sold his house to the nonprofit service organization. In this way residents could have Japanese-speaking aides, Japanese-style cuisine, and feel comfortable conversing freely with other residents who share their cultural background. Other Asian groups have also developed board and cares for their elderly populations. Even though the tradition of strong family relationships is a part of their respective cultures, because of the social differences in the United States which seem to undermine the extended kinship settlements of their native lands, they, too, have looked upon board and cares as an attractive housing choice. At the time this Japanese home was being developed, a German-speaking organization and a Jewish group contacted the Japanese board and care operator to inquire how the program started.

The Jewish community has for many years developed residences across the nation for elders. Homes for Jewish parents are situated in many localities. The elderly inhabitants can speak to one another in Yiddish or Hebrew, eat kosher foods if they like, celebrate special religious holidays and ceremonies, and remain safe from the anti-Semitism they may have experienced in the "outside" world. Such an environment can have enormous appeal for orthodox Jews.

Many metropolitan areas are rich with a diverse array of cultural and ethnic groups, and many of their organizations have built senior residences. The San Francisco Bay Area is no exception. In the East Bay, with its substantial African-American population, a number of church-related residences provide housing for elders: for example, the Allen Temple Arms, associated with the Allen Temple Baptist Church in Oakland; and the Harriet Tubman Terrace in Berkeley, an HUD-financed retirement complex. This doesn't mean that only African-Americans live in these homes. On the contrary, they are represented in other facilities as well as church-related homes, union-affiliated residences, and larger retirement complexes. For some, the choice is determined by the desire to share a common religion; for others, cost is the determining factor; while for still others, it may be the need to live near friends. There are many reasons for choosing to live in senior board and care housing.

Shared interests and cultural heritage do make for comfortable living arrangements, especially when elders feel physically and/or socially vulnerable. For example, an Hispanic man living in a board and care where no one spoke his native language, kept asking for something but no one could understand what he wanted. It turned out that all he wanted was some Mexican food. "Anyone could have walked down a couple of blocks and brought him a taco or enchilada," said the staff member who related the story. Instead, the man was categorized as a "troublesome patient" and pushed aside. It is easy to see why elders with special language preferences would want caregivers who can speak to them in their native tongue.

Board and cares have grown to meet the needs of elders who can no longer live alone. For most older people and their (remaining) family members, safety—both from outside assault and from their own confusion and disabilities—makes the board and care a viable alternative living arrangement. Next we will look at the general profile of board and care residents and those who are likely to benefit from the services these residential care facilities provide.

WHO RESIDES IN BOARD AND CARES?

The vast majority of board and care residents are older adults who cannot live safely on their own at home, yet they do not require full-time skilled nursing care. These persons may be mentally impaired or confused; developmentally disabled (and in need of learning or relearning personal, social, or interpersonal skills); victims of stroke, heart attack, or some other disabling illness or accident. Our general profile of elderly board and care residents shows the following:

(1) They can no longer live safely at home on their own, and in many cases they are no longer able to fully satisfy their own needs.

(2) Many are single or, if widowed, have outlived one or more spouses—some have even outlived their own children.

(3) They have more than one physical or mental impairment. Confusion is a major reason for their inability to live in safety by themselves in their own homes. For example, an older person might turn on the stove or a water faucet and forget about it. Others may go out for a walk and forget how to get home.

(4) Their income is too low to enable them to live in a "life care"-type of retirement complex. (Life care implies room, meals, education and/or recreation opportunities, medical supervision, and intermediate or full-time skilled nursing care for as long a the person lives.)

(5) Some older adults may need some help but are alert and prefer to live in their own neighborhood instead of moving to unfamiliar surroundings. Familiar neighborhoods are especially important to elders who may be slightly confused.

(6) They require some help with activities of daily living, such as money management and transportation assistance.

(7) Some have a major chronic and/or disabling condition (e.g., the effects of a stroke, Acquired Immune Deficiency Syndrome, heart attack, severe arthritis, or cancer) but remain mentally alert and ambulatory. They can follow their doctor's instructions without supervision.

(8) For others, either their families don't want to care for them or feel they can't provide the kind of care needed. (The elder may want more attention than the family is prepared or able to give; confusion makes the elderly relative a danger; or the family's activities will be significantly curtailed as a result of the need for someone to remain with the aged person.)

In March 1990, the editor of the *Continuing Care Resources* newsletter mentioned a study that discussed other characteristics of board and care residents. We list several below that are of particular interest:

(1) On the average, board and care residents are in their mid to late eighties. Over the past few years the average age has been increasing. (At Salem, in 1989, there were twenty-five residents over ninety years of age.)

(2) Most residents have led a relatively normal, ordinary life—i.e., career, marriage, and children.

(3) Almost all residents entered board and cares near the end of their lives. For many, unless they require more intense levels of care, this will be their home for the rest of their lives.[4]

We harbor no illusions that the above list covers all pertinent characteristics of those who make board and care facilities their home, but it should provide some idea of who the residents are. Our list was developed from information we have gathered over the years in our respective careers. The list of services that should be made available to board and care residents is provided below. Once these essential services are outlined, a better picture emerges of why this kind of living arrangement suits so many elders.

WHAT KINDS OF SERVICES DO
BOARD AND CARE RESIDENTS NEED?

If older adults are to manage in the board and care setting, many support services are needed that will enable them to perform their ordinary activities of daily living and instrumental activities of daily living. The former include such services as offering assistance in walking, bathing, dressing, and transferring (from bed to chair, from chair to toilet, etc.). Instrumental activities may include doing laundry, making a telephone call, shopping, assistance in taking medicines (both the prescribed dosage and at the designated time), money management, and housework. Thus, elders may need some or all of the following services:

(1) *Meal Preparation:* Elders who live alone often say "It's too much trouble to cook for myself, so I don't eat much any more." As mental or physical disability sets in, cooking might become dangerous, shopping for food is ignored, reduced feelings of hunger are experienced, or meals are no longer prepared. At board and care homes, well-balanced meals can be prepared and served at regular times. Good nutrition is important at any age.

(2) *Personal Care:* This may include help with bathing (getting in and out of tubs or showers); selecting appropriate clothes and helping residents dress for the day; grooming hair, nails, and face; toileting or changing undergarments for incontinent persons.

(3) *Laundry Service:* Staff is provided to wash linens (sheets, towels, etc.) and/or residents' personal clothing items.

(4) *Transportation:* Car or van service is provided to residents so they can go to the store or see to medical appointments. Sometimes taxi-scripts are provided to elder residents. A board and care facility will make special arrangements with a local taxi service to transport residents at affordable rates.

(5) *Escort Services:* Some elders are *physically* able to use public transportation or call a taxi, but due to their confused state, they are unable depart for and return from their appointments alone. These older persons may have gone to the same doctor's office for many years and know the location by heart, but, after exiting a bus or cab, they forget which way to go. Others may be able to give their cab driver an address, but unless the driver helps them out

of the cab and into the building, they may not be able to reach their final destination.

For these elders, an escort service is very important. If a cab driver lets them off on the sidewalk and leaves without pointing them in the right direction, they may wander aimlessly for a long time—a dangerous situation. Even for those who are in good mental health, it is easy to become disoriented in an unfamiliar place. But for the confused elder, it can be both difficult and frightening when street noises and the movements of strangers add to their sense of uncertainty. Sometimes panic sets in. Escort services provide helpful people who ensure that the elders reach their intended destination and return safely to the board and care facility.

(6) *Activities:* Residents are provided with creative ways to occupy their time and to stimulate their senses as well as their mental abilities. These activities are designed to help them maintain a healthy level of mental, physical, spiritual, and emotional well-being.

(7) *Socialization Opportunities:* Residents are provided with experiences that allow them to expand and sharpen their interpersonal skills. Advancing age should not be an obstacle to continued social interaction. These opportunities can take the form of casual daily coffee hours, or involve more structured events such as trips, parties, outings to community events, dances, and much more.

Board and care homes do not supervise medication. Lacking the services of a registered nurse, they are not responsible for administering medicines. However, this restriction does not preclude board and care staff from knowing when medications must be taken and then encouraging the resident(s) to take them appropriately. Anything more than basic encouragement would fall under the purview of functions performed by nursing homes, which do regulate the flow of medications. Board and care workers may, of course, place medications at the meal table or remind residents to take their prescriptions at specified times. If a resident reaches the point at which regular nursing care is needed, the physician of record should consider transferring the individual to a skilled nursing facility.

MANDATED ACTIVITIES FOR BOARD AND CARE LICENSING

Unfortunately, there have been problems in the board and care field, as in any industry. Mismanagement, incompetence, and outright exploitation have occurred. In the past two decades federal attempts have been made to protect board and care residents. The 1976 Keys Amendment to the Social Security Act required each state to establish standards for residential care facilities. Homes found not to comply with existing state standards would experience the reduction of SSI payments to residents in their charge, and hence a reduction of their own income. Then in 1981 the Rinaldo Amendment to the Older Americans Act placed board and cares under the blanket protection of each states Long-Term Care Ombudsman Program. The office of ombudsman serves as a conduit for information to and from residents, families, and caregivers, as well as federal and state agencies. The goal of the ombudsman is to assist all parties in resolving problems that arise and to improve the well-being of elders by protecting their interests.

Though such federal legislation has been instrumental in improving the lives of board and care residents throughout the country, much remains to be done. One such area is activities to stimulate and revitalize residents in the hope that improved levels of mental and physical capacity and endurance will significantly reduce the amount of custodial care needed. This particular area of concern does not fall under the jurisdiction of federal legislation pertaining to the elderly or to programs affecting them. For this reason, we must turn to the states for guidance with respect to innovative legislation.

According to the Adult Residential Licensing regulations of the State of California, "The Licensee shall insure that planned recreational activities which include the following are provided for their clients:

(1) Activities that require group interaction;

(2) Physical activities—including but not limited to games, sports, and exercises;

(3) In facilities with a licensed capacity of 50 or more clients, a current, written program of activities shall be planned in advance and made available to all clients;

(4) Activities shall be encouraged through provision of space, equipment, and supplies. . . ."[5]

The above types of activities are part of California's licensing requirements contained in Title 22 covering Residential Care Facilities for the Elderly. A significant portion of this book contains instructions for activities that will help board and care owners and operators fill these requirements or similar licensing regulations of other states.

Board and cares do more than provide some or all of the direct services listed above. They also serve as a link between residents and service providers in the community at large, some of which transport residents to Social Day Care Centers for interaction with other people, for meals at local nutrition sites, for adult day health-care services, for educational or recreational classes or for exercise programs, and for social events in the community. Arrangements can be made with churches, synagogues, civic groups, senior citizens centers, and others to come pick up residents for services or other special programs. This gives the elders a continuing involvement in their church and a chance to see long-time friends. Through volunteer programs like Friendly Visitors* or telephone assurance groups, board and cares can arrange outside visits from volunteers for residents who no longer have relatives to come see them. In this way these older persons continue to feel that someone "out there" cares about them. The importance of these kinds of community contacts for the mental and physical well-being of elders who have limited mobility can never be overemphasized.

A FINANCIAL PROFILE OF BOARD AND CARE RESIDENTS

Studies show that as many as 80 percent of the elders who live in board and cares depend primarily on Social Security for the majority of their income. Most rely on Supplementary Security Income (SSI) or Social Security Disability Income (SSDI) as their sole source of income, but these funds barely cover monthly fees. Many board and cares are required by law to guarantee their residents that 10 percent of the elders' total income will be available as private spending money. Out of this amount, residents are expected to buy personal care items such as lotions, cosmetics or hair preparations, snacks, gifts or cards, stationery, or toothpaste. It is important for elders who have lost so much control over their lives to be able to have some say in how their money is spent. What may appear to many to be simple, almost insignificant actions or choices give

---

*For information on one form of a "Friendly Visitors" program, readers are directed to Appendix 8.

older people a valued sense of personal control and a feeling of individual dignity.

Residents who have relatives, children, or close friends may at times receive gifts of personal items, clothing, or even money. These gifts help tremendously and are very welcome, but it is important to realize that the elderly want to reciprocate in some manner, even though their lack of funds makes this very difficult. The lack of adequate income and spending money also limits the number of "outside" events some residents can attend— e.g., ball games, concerts, shows, and shopping excursions. We are not saying that all residents of board and cares are plagued by low income, but for a large number of today's elderly, income is an important consideration and a constant source of concern.

Because residents' income levels are generally low and the rate of federal and state reimbursement to board and cares is also low, the quality of care that residents receive is adversely affected. California State Senator Nicholas Petris, who has introduced a number of bills in the state legislature to improve the lives of elders, has said that operators contend that they do not make enough profit from board and cares to offer much beyond basic services. It would seem, then, that we need to advocate for adequate reimbursement to operators, whether the funds come from Medicare, Medicaid, Social Security, or private insurance. Federal and state budget cuts may exacerbate an already painful situation among those who operate the nation's board and care facilities. Clearly one significant advantage for residents would be to require that insurance plans pay for rent and services, provided, of course, it can be established that to do so would be far less costly than placing the individual in a skilled nursing facility. We suspect that the savings would certainly substantiate the need for a change in policy.

QUALITY OF CARE

The phrase "quality of care" is widely used when referring to services provided to the elderly. Exactly what do we mean by quality of care? We use the phrase to mean health-enhancing environments and services that add to an individual's well-being. In particular we mean it to apply to the lives of those who are no longer able to manage their own activities of daily living. This may include getting well-prepared, good-tasting, nutritionally balanced meals that are appetizing and attractively served; opportunities to have stimulating activities that help the elders maintain good mental and physical health; regularly scheduled religious or spiritual programs if the residents want them; and frequent occasions for socializing. In the Winter 1989 issue of the American Society on Aging's publication *Generations,* guest editor Robert Applebaum discusses ways in which "quality of care" can be assured. He suggests that "persons who receive good levels of care get benefits and happiness from receiving them, and that the services are doing what they are supposed to do. Also, that elders who receive these services are better off than those who do not have access to similar services."[6]

Conversely, then, poor quality of care would include unsatisfactory services that fail to achieve their intended purposes; in other words, they create or aggravate unsatisfactory living environments (e.g., dirty floors, dusty or poorly ventilated rooms, dull food, poor lighting, lax safety precautions, etc.) as well as a lack of stimulating activities and socialization opportunities to help maintain a good level of mental and physical health. Even if basic meals, a place to sleep, and some personal care services are provided, these do not necessarily mean that a good quality of care has been offered.

The meaning of quality of care can be appreciated through the experiences of members of the Berkeley California Chapter of Gray Panthers, who in 1982 began studying the need for changes in the long-term care given to residents of nursing homes. Many of these advocates for the elderly were surprised when people heard about the aims of their group and started coming to meetings to share experiences. At one meeting, a woman told about the plight of her mother, who had spent what assets she had to stay in a private nursing home. She then had to move to a less expensive public facility. A man recounted his efforts to get a nursing facility's staff to walk with his wife on the days when he could not be there, so that she would remain mobile. They didn't and she deteriorated rapidly.

In our professional experience, we have seen other elderly parents placed in nursing homes even though they were able to manage quite a few of their activities of daily living. For example, one woman was placed in a skilled nursing facility because her children did not feel that they could take care of her themselves, but together they were able to pay the costs of keeping her in the nursing home. Though she experienced partial impairment as a result of a stroke—she needed help with bathing and transferring to bed—the woman could take her medicines and could walk to various activities. She was able to embroider and engage in other craft activities, played table games with other residents, and, in our opinion, did not belong in a full-time skilled nursing facility. If a board and care had been readily available and had the family known of it, this woman would have been an ideal candidate.

Evaluating quality of care is difficult. There are many board and care facilities in California: some are good, some are not. In our experience, the great majority of board and cares we know of do try very hard to provide basic care at a level satisfactory to all residents. However, according to investigations made by the staff of the Little Hoover Commission: "The historical record of Board and Cares is fraught with abuse and neglect of their elderly residents including mismanagement and violations of their [the operator's] licensing requirements."[7]*

California State Senator Petris told us that operators voice to him their frustration that reimbursement rates are so low that they can barely provide more than minimal care. Board and care operators say that Medicare-Medicaid reimbursements for services do not cover the hiring of extra staff or persons who are trained to lead activities that stimulate the mental and physical health of their residents. The operators also told him they feel that the whole licensing process and requirements are harrowing, cumbersome, and costly. It would seem that even efforts designed to help make the system more efficient do not always result in the hoped for benefits. In addition to the Keys Amendment, which forced states to pass bills requiring minimum standards in all board and cares over which they exercise jurisdiction, some states have gone so far as to introduce laws requiring board and care operators to take specific training courses. It appears, then, that many people are concerned about the quality of care given to residents in board and care homes, especially as these facilities gain popularity as a cost-effective housing and care alternative for many of our nation's elders.

CAREGIVERS

The primary caregiving staff of board and cares may not face the twenty-four-hour job that family caregivers do, but the work is hard, often emotionally draining, and poorly compensated—barely minimum wage in most cases. The staff needs continuous, on-the-job training and counseling. How does this relate to the issue of quality of care? Again and again,

---

*This statement seems to focus on licensed residential facilities only. There are many board and cares accommodating so few residents/clients that they are too small to require a license.

as we listened to the people who came to committee meetings for nursing home reform, we were made aware of how important the issue of quality of care is to elderly residents of board and cares. It is important both to their wellness and to the families' sense of security that their relatives are receiving the best possible care.

Recently, a number of very elderly Japanese-speaking persons were interviewed by Ivy Down. The one quality they all felt was most important in a caregiver was what they called *shinsetsu,* a term that incorporates the Chinese character for "heart" or "spirit." These elders wanted a caring person. Employees can be trained with specific job skills, but the quality of being sensitive and caring toward persons who are among society's most vulnerable is an important one that is not easily instilled.

A man whose elderly female relative lives in a nursing home described a problem employee. He said that a frustrated aide was using crude and abusive language toward his loved one: the person with whom she shared a room was incontinent and needed her clothes changed frequently, which upset the aide. Although this happened in a nursing home, similar care needs are handled by board and care aides. This example is used to illustrate the kind of hard and often disagreeable work these aides perform: the heavy lifting involved in transferring or otherwise moving a resident, cleaning up after those who have toileting accidents, the emotional stress of daily work with frail and often confused older people. If the aide mentioned above had received the training needed to more effectively handle such situations, and counseling to cope with the stress of a demanding workload, she would not have expressed frustration toward the resident's room-mate. If training and counseling do not help alleviate staff-resident conflicts, then abusive employees should be transferred to different jobs in which direct contact with residents is minimized.* Certainly, quality of care goes hand in hand with well-trained, sensitive caregivers.

HOW CAN QUALITY OF CARE BE IMPROVED?

When board and care operators are adequately licensed, monitored, and reimbursed, and when they are encouraged to offer the types and levels of care needed by their residents, then we will begin to see a good quality of care developing throughout the industry. Conversely, operators of poorly

---

*In such cases family members may wish to consult the long-term care ombudsman to prevent such incidents from being repeated.

managed, abusive, or neglectful facilities must be held accountable for their treatment of the elderly, and, when infractions occur, they should be prosecuted to the fullest extent of the law.

Our observations and diverse experiences with regard to board and cares or similar residential care facilities suggest to us that quality care should include the following:

(1) *Better training for all staff persons* who directly care for residents (aides, housekeepers, cooks and kitchen help, and the administrators who supervise them; caregivers who work directly with residents; and various support groups). These caregivers are most often the people best able both to determine and directly affect the quality of care that board and care clients receive.

(2) *Adequate pay.* Given the physical demands of their work, the emotional stress, the levels of care to be provided, the patience needed to perform these tasks, and the restraint that the caregivers must constantly exercise, board and care employees deserve adequate pay. The scale that currently exists will continue to result in employee dissatisfaction and high turnover rates. Impaired elders, many of whom require a very structured environment, find it hard to cope with a steady flow of unfamiliar staff members who must learn the daily routine anew. Significant turnover in staff can be very unsettling for residents, many of whom stand to suffer when the level of care is diminished as a result.

(3) *Uniform standards* of care and basic licensing requirements are vital. Should there be some nationwide basic standard for board and cares or residential facilities, with clearly defined minimum levels of care? Currently there is a great diversity among various types of facilities in each of the fifty states: an uneven reimbursement pattern, widely divergent levels of care available to residents, and varying levels of supervision or monitoring. Still, it does seem possible to develop simple, basic health regulations that can be established on the national level but supervised and monitored by existing state regulatory agencies (e.g., health departments, social service agencies, adult protective services, etc.). As the number of board and cares continues to grow, the need for a federal supervisory agency—if not federal legislation—becomes ever more urgent.

Ensuring good, quality care may not be easy. Board and care operators will need incentives to provide it. For a more in-depth understanding of the issue of quality care, readers are directed to the Winter 1989 issue of the American Society on Aging's publication *Generations,* which focuses on "Assuring Quality of Care." Dr. Robert Applebaum, in an article written for the same issue, states that "quality assurance asks the following questions:

> (1) Does the service match the practice standards that have been identified,
>
> and
>
> (2) is the service being provided in the way that it was developed?"[8]

He goes on to say,

> Thus, quality is defined as "conformation to requirements" and quality assurance is the set of methods used to create, reinforce and maintain this conformance. Overall, combining practice standards (knowing what the intervention is), program evaluation (knowing the outcomes of a service), and quality assurance (knowing that the service is implemented in a consistent manner as designed) results in the ability to provide high quality of care.[9]

Dr. Applebaum asserts that if quality assurance standards are set and maintained, it will be possible to design a standard of quality by which board and cares can be evaluated. Perhaps then, we can even develop a level of accountability for operators to strive for and maintain.

In the same issue of *Generations,* Dr. Charles Sabatino, Assistant Director for the Council on Legal Problems of the Elderly, in Washington, D.C., discusses how a program for accountability among board and care operators might be developed.

> Many different groups are working innovatively on these various fronts . . . (but are) still far from the goal of achieving a coherent system of accountability.
>
> Some existing vehicles for accountability are:
>
> (1) voluntary accreditation and licensure;
> (2) client empowerment and involvement with residents involved from the beginning in planning, program evaluation, monitoring, and enforcement which includes
>> (a) a client grievance process and ombudsman program;
>> (b) peer review organizations;

       (c) the State's role in monitoring and enforcement with power to enforce sanctions such as fines or refusing to renew licensing. The last (c) State's role only applies to Medicare/Medicaid-covered home care.[10]

On the other hand, Jan Chernak of Hillhaven Corporation, which owns a large chain of nursing homes, credits her program with maintaining a high quality of care. "Care is taken to assure that the program incorporates practices as required by law while also adhering to standards set by the Joint Commission on Accreditation of Hospitals. The Program also depends on the cooperation and resourcefulness of its facilities. The heart of the program is the 'Quality Assurance Committee' at each facility, which monitors infection control, utilization reviews, resident/staff safety, and [committees of residents] which routinely participate in monitoring overall patient care."[11] Under the watchful eye of such committees, Hillhaven's facilities maintain a good level of care.

In an article for the same Winter 1989 issue of *Generations,* Rosalie A. and Robert L. Kane address the question of quality control. More specifically, they concentrate on the many difficulties that can arise when trying to set up scientific measurements to quantify quality of care, including the reality that what works well for one older person may not benefit another elder who appears to have similar ailments. The Kanes point out that this need for individualized care sometimes "makes it hard to define goals . . . and highly desirable goals may often be impossible to achieve simultaneously, for example, cognitive functioning [memory, awareness, and reasoning] is worsened by drugs that relieve pain."[12]

Professionals who have worked toward a nationwide standard of quality care acknowledge that achieving this admirable goal requires caregivers and advocates of the elderly to address many complex and multifaceted issues. The number of concerns—some specific, others more general—that confront those who attempt to construct and implement such a standard are considerable. Yet, since quality of care is important (and in conversations with residents and their families it comes through loud and clear as the paramount concern), then studies and systems like the ones just mentioned will help all concerned to ensure and to enforce a good quality of care among all board and care providers.

NOTES

1. The American Association of Retired Persons, *A Home Away From Home: Consumer Information on Board and Care Homes* (Washington, D.C.: The American Association of Retired Persons, Consumer Affairs, 1988).

2. "Newsbriefs," in the American Society on Aging bimonthly newspaper *The Aging Connection* (February/March, 1990).

3. Marilyn Moon, "Introduction," in *Preserving Independence, Supporting Needs: The Role of Board and Care Homes,* edited by Marilyn Moon, George Gaberlavage, and Sandra J. Newman (Washington, D.C.: Public Policy Institute, American Association of Retired Persons, 1989), p. viii.

4. Shelagh Nebocat, ed., *Continuing Care Resources* (South Burnaby, British Columbia, Canada: Amour Health Associates, Ltd.). The study was conducted by Eileen Garvey of the Pearson Center and Association of Extended Care Units.

5. "Operating Without a License," California State Regulations on Community Care License Requirements, CARCH News (March 1988):17-19.

6. Robert Applebaum, "What's All This About Quality?" *Generations,* special issue on Assuring Quality of Care (Winter 1989):5-7.

7. Little Hoover Commission public hearing, State of California Legislature, Friday, April 29, 1988, in San Francisco.

8. Applebaum, "What's All This About Quality?"

9. Ibid.

10. Charles Sabatino, "Putting Public Accountability to the Test," *Generations* (Winter 1989):12-16.

11. Jan Chernak (Vice President, Hillhaven Corporation, Quality Assurance Plan), "Providing Quality Care Isn't Enough Anymore," *Generations* (Winter 1989):60, 62.

12. Rosalie A. Kane and Robert L. Kane, "Reflections on Quality Control," *Generations* (Winter 1989):63-68.

RESOURCES

Readers concerned about issues pertaining to quality of care should write or call:

> *Generations*
> c/o The American Society on Aging
> 833 Market Street, Rm 516
> San Francisco, CA 94103
> (415) 543-2617

to order a copy of the Winter 1989 issue. It contains seventeen articles on various aspects of quality of care. Public libraries or your local Area Agency on Aging may also have a copy of this valuable publication.

In addition to the literature and agencies discussed in this chapter, organizations such as

Ombudsman, Inc.
Citizens Serving Long-Term Care Residents
1212 Broadway, Suite 606
Oakland, CA 94612-1824
(510) 465-1065

provide volunteers who go into long-term care facilities to determine that residents are not only receiving the services to which they are entitled, but also that they receive quality care. Direct services offered by this group include:

- weekly visits to assigned nursing homes and residential care facilities;
- receiving and resolving complains, misunderstandings, and grievances from residents and/or their families;
- monitoring the quality of care that residents receive;
- solving problems having to do with meals, finances, health-related issues, theft, or other personal difficulties residents experience;
- being a witness for Durable Power of Attorney for health care, wills, natural death directives, transfer of property, and any other needed witnessing.

State and local ombudsmen provide families with such valuable information as the cost of care at various facilities, how to select a care facility, or suggestions about where concerned relatives or elders can go for help with specific questions that may be beyond the ombudsman's expertise.

Publications provided by organizations like Ombudsman, Inc., include:

"How to Choose a Nursing Home,"
"List of Residential Care and Skilled Licensed Nursing Homes,"
"Observation List for Skilled Nursing Homes,"
"Things You Should Know When Entering a Nursing Home,"
"Choices When Help Is Needed in Managing Affairs,"
"Supplemental Security Income, Med-Cal, Medicare,"
"Observation List for Nursing Facilities."

The ombudsman nearest you can be located by contacting your State Long-Term Care Ombudsman office. A list of state offices is provided in Appendix 5.

2

Case Management

Most people can describe, in basic terms, how doctors and nurses interact within a residential care facility, and many can outline some of the functions that these professionals perform. But less well known is the work of another health-care professional, a person who operates behind the scenes to coordinate the many different kinds of treatment, resources, and services that go into good care. This person, known as a case manager, may be a social worker, a nurse, a gerontologist, a counselor, a paraprofessional, and in some cases just a family member. Case managers are found in a variety of settings: nursing homes, hospitals, health maintenance organizations (HMOs), government organizations, the private sector, and residential care facilities for elders (board and cares).

WHAT IS CASE MANAGEMENT?

Case management is the art of overseeing the many aspects of a resident's life. For the board and care residents, the case manager ensures that certain medical, dental, nutritional, and social service needs are met expediently. Individual social service needs may include finding money management services, making sure that "Friendly Visitors," are available to residents on an "as-needed" basis, and helping to provide supplies that ensure personal hygiene. Family members will probably meet their relatives' case manager during the initial care planning process or during visits to the board and care facility. Families should always feel free to ask the case manager any questions pertaining to the care and treatment of their loved one.

After questioning the case manager, Mrs. J.'s family, for example, wanted to know if she could get taxi script to visit them on Sundays. Mrs. J. required renal dialysis and must have regular treatment three times each week. She is slowly adjusting to life at the board and care, but she is not able to make friends easily. Mrs. J.'s family was relieved to know that she did qualify for the taxi script program.

Even in situations where board and cares are offering appropriate basic services, more effort and coordination of these services may be needed in order to ensure that residents can remain stabilized for as long as possible. Often case management services can forestall the mental and/or physical deterioration that so often results from nursing home placement. Thus, some facilities employ a case manager hoping that, with close monitoring, their residents will be able to remain part of the board and care family for a much longer period of time.

According to one expert, case management "is a fluid process which includes client assessment and the provision, coordination and monitoring of services."[1] The process remains fluid because the various needs of residents change over time. For example, an elder who enters a board and care in reasonable good health or in a stable condition may become physically ill or mentally confused, thereby requiring a different level of care than other residents in the same facility. In other cases, illnesses that had been controlled quite well with prescribed medications may suddenly become more severe and medical assessment may reveal a need to explore or change dosage or possibly prescribe new medicine. Then again, some residents who are quite alert and rational when they first enter a board and care may, after a period of time, start to mimic the confused or chaotic behavior of other residents in the facility. While board and care owners/ managers may not be skilled enough to recognize these changes, a case manager is trained to watch for them.

Growing old is not easy. Whether an elder lives independently, stays with relatives, or resides at a board and care, urinary incontinence can be a serious and pervasive problem. Clothing is damaged, the person is often embarrassed, activities are restricted, and one's general quality of life deteriorates unless measures are taken. The case manager can see to it that the elder is supplied with the appropriate personal care products and coached on how to use them. In addition, the case manager can recommend counseling to help affected persons regain their self-esteem and confidence. A case manager can help in a number of ways: educating residents regarding toileting regimes, securing a consultation with a physical therapist about exercises to improve bladder control and strengthen bladder muscles, and assessing the kinds and quantities of incontinency aids needed and where they can be acquired. In some facilities the case manager may even need to be involved with suppliers of incontinency aids to assure on-time delivery of these much-needed products.

THE ROLE OF THE CASE MANAGER

The role of the case manager in a board and care or residential care setting can give new meaning to creative case management. New approaches to solving old problems are sought and implemented. Long-established attitudes and practices are often challenged and changed. For example, case managers may challenge the belief that resident elders need little more than a safe place to stay and basic care for the rest of their natural lives. The very idea that the aged need to continue exercising their minds and bodies and to maintain as high a level of interaction with their former community and friends as possible is certainly a revolutionary thought. Exploring new avenues for meeting the needs of residents can appear threatening to managers, especially if they are expected to implement new policies and practices on their own. A case manager, on the other hand, is skilled in handling clients, and realizes that changes can be unsettling. Change can be implemented in ways that reduce fear and anxiety on the part of both board and care managers and residents. Examples can be found in the case of Mrs. F. who is deaf and needs encouragement to interact more with hearing residents, or Mr. M. for whom certain types of food are culturally unfamiliar.

For the last five years Lorraine Schnurr has worked as part of a case management team in the community and in twelve board and cares in Oakland, California. She works in the Multipurpose Senior Services Program (MSSP) and in a separate MSSP-sponsored project called the "Community Care Facilities for the Elderly" (CCFE) demonstration project, which provides case management services to the board and cares.

MSSP operates under the auspices of the City of Oakland's Office on Aging and is an eleven-year-old long-term care program designed to keep elders from premature institutionalization. CCFE and MSSP receive multiple funding, which includes Medicaid waivers (called MediCal waivers in California) from the Federal Health Care Financing Administration. Participants in the MSSP and CCFE programs must meet the following eligibility requirements:

- be sixty-five years of age or older;

- live in Oakland, California;

- be certifiable for a skilled nursing (SNF) or intermediate care facility (ICF);

- have Medi-Cal coverage without a share of the cost.

These two programs must be cost effective, that is, the cost of keeping elders in the community or in the board and care must be less than the cost of care in a SNF or ICF. Being "certifiable" means that the residents' physical and mental conditions are such that the individuals would qualify for placement in an ICF or SNF. Residents most likely to be certified by a physican for skilled or intermediate nursing facilities are those who need twenty-four-hour nursing care.

As a case manager for the community-based Senior Services program and for the demonstration project at board and cares, it has been Lorraine's job to screen and assess elderly clients, develop care plans, order and monitor the services provided to clients, reassess elderly clients at regular intervals, and advocate on behalf of board and care residents as well as various other older adults who live independently in the community. Being involved in case management at both a community program and a board and care project has given her a unique opportunity to compare and contrast both the CCFE and MSSP. The needs of board and care residents are different from elderly persons living in the community, and the services to meet those needs must also be different.

Differing Needs of Elders in the Community and Those in Board and Cares

An elderly person struggling to remain independent may need a combination of services: domestic help, personal care, low-cost housing, home-delivered meals, minor home repairs, home safety checks, or legal services. On the other hand, a board and care resident may need only additional help with personal care and money management or assistance in securing a payee representative or a conservator to remain in a board and care. We assume that the basic services of meal preparation, housing, transportation, housekeeping, social interaction, and supervision in a semi-protected environment are already being met by the residential facility.

Another difference between the CCFE and the MSSP is the number and frequency of visits to clients in each setting. According to guidelines set by the California State Department on Aging, board and care clients must be seen monthly, while community-based clients are visited quarterly. Lorraine has observed that, when compared to elders living in the community, board and care residents are diagnosed with more dementia. Many are confused and require longer visits. Furthermore, the only allowable service purchased, via medical waivers, for these clients is additional personal care assistance. It is not the intention of the CCFE to supplant services that board and care staff members are already providing. Additional personal care service can be given to residents who need more help with bathing, grooming, toileting, feeding, and dressing, which is above and beyond what the staff already provides. Personal care also includes other activities such as bowel and bladder training, reality orientation,* socialization, light massage to increase circulation, and help to move about within the facility.

Services that clients receive are either purchased, referred, or provided by friends or family. Purchased services for both the CCFE and the MSSP are contracted from an agency in the community which is accountable to the MSSP. There must be at least five residents in the board and care facility before these services can be provided on a contract basis. It is simply more cost-effective for a nursing assistant to provide services to a group of five as opposed to a smaller number of residents.

Elderly clients living in their own homes or with relatives may have a wide variety of "purchased services" available to them:

- adult social day care

- nonmedical equipment (equipment not covered by Medicare, Medicaid, or medical insurance)

- skilled nursing care

- transportation

- minor home repair

- domestic and personal care

- translation services

- food supplements

---

*Assessing residents' ability to know and recall their own names, where they live, the time of day, day of week and month, the names of significant others, and related questions that assist in determining levels of mental confusion.

Referred services are those paid for by MediCal, Medicaid, or Medicare dollars, and include the following:

- medical equipment and supplies
- inpatient and outpatient hospital services
- physician/dental services and medications
- medical transportation.

If a board and care resident needs to attend an adult day health-care center, a referral would be made to an agency that provides the service. If a resident needs transportation to go grocery shopping, the case manager might refer the client to a service that would meet that need. There are times when a case manager cannot purchase services or refer a client to an existing service. For example, Mr. J. lives in a board and care and is unable to speak English. The case manager may have to secure translation services informally through a volunteer from a local church.

It is often difficult to provide services to board and care residents because many more people with an interest in the client's well-being get involved. This group may include the board and care manager, the resident, a vendor responsible for supervising the staff person assigned to the board and care, family members, conservators, and/or a state licensing department analyst. Arranging a conference with all of these people can be extremely time consuming.

For example, it was 6 P.M. before all of the interested persons involved in Mr. F.'s care could be assembled to discuss his move from Oakland to a hospital in San Francisco. Although Mr. F. had no family members, his conservator, the board and care operator, the case manager, and his certified nursing assistant were all present at the conference to offer immediate input and to make tentative plans for Mr. F.'s return from the hospital. Mr. F.'s primary care physician was located in San Francisco, and the California State Licensing analyst was concerned about Mr. F.'s present weakened condition as well as his inability to walk from his bed to the chair in his room. Mr. F.'s prospects for remaining in the board and care were at issue.

Finally, the different needs of clients in the community as compared to those in board and cares changes the care-planning process in each group. Making a care plan for the community-based elder may involve different purchased and referred services, all of which have to be monitored.

A care plan for board and care residents may require that only one additional "purchased service" be monitored. Nonetheless, care plans for CCFE and MSSP participants involve the same basic steps. Yet, more advocacy and education (of management, staff, residents, and their families) may be needed in the board and care setting.

STEPS IN CASE MANAGEMENT

Effective case management on the board and care level involves many elements if quality care is to meet residents' needs:

(1) *Screening:* This is the initial process whereby the prospective client is evaluated for CCFE/MSSP services. Criteria for eligibility include age, income, residence, cost effectiveness, health status, financial ability, recent hospitalizations, cognitive ability, and social support in the community. Screening is a valuable preliminary step before a lengthy, full assessment is embarked upon by the case management team. For those persons who are not old enough, who live outside of the service area, who have no functional limitations, or who otherwise do not fit the criteria, the screener may be able to suggest other resources and/or services in the community.

(2) *Assessment:* If the client is passed through the preliminary screening, a second evaluation is done in the client's home to assess physical and mental functioning, social networks, financial resources, past medical history, present medical condition, and current medications. The team also asks about present use of available resources: Is the client already attending a social day-care program? Is he or she receiving home-delivered meals or using subsidized transportation? Is the client involved with a local church? Since Lorraine and Ivy are particularly interested in sensory losses experienced by board and care residents, Lorraine conducts informal assessments of how well clients can see, hear, smell, taste, or touch according to self-reports or available medical information. These data are extremely important for planning meaningful social activities that board and care residents can participate in.

(3) *Care Plan Development:* A tailor-made plan is developed by an elder care team composed of a nurse, a social worker, and a supervising case manager. Either the nurse or the social worker can have primary responsibility for a particular client. The findings of these professionals are combined with input from the client. Other individuals who often provide input for the care plan process are: family members, gerontologists, medical staff professionals, friends and unrelated significant others, and the board and care staff who will actually provide services to the residents. After the problems are identified, the care plan becomes a "road map" of *what* needs to be done and *who* is assigned to perform which tasks.

(4) *Purchase or Referral of Services:* This phase of case management involves the process of securing the actual services clients need if they are to remain in the community or in a board and care setting. Services are purchased from several outside vendors who are under contract with the City of Oakland's MSSP/CCFE Program. Referred services are paid for through Medicaid/MediCal or Medicare and include adult day health care as well as social day-care programs, medical, dental, podiatry, and legal services.

(5) *Monitoring Services:* After services have been purchased or referred, the case manager then has to make sure that the services or supplies have been delivered in a satisfactory and timely manner and are being utilized. CCFE monitoring involves mandated monthly visits, assessing the quality of the services being delivered, and informally determining the degree of satisfaction with the services provided. Some key questions often asked by case manager are:

- Is the service adequate?

- What is the quality of the service?

- Does the client need something more?

- Is there an obstacle preventing the client from using the service?

The monitoring of both board and care and community services can be conducted by telephone to clients, during home visits, or by reading vendor reports.

(6) *Reassessment:* The case manager assesses the needs of clients on an on-going basis. This is essential to assure that levels of service remain consistent with client needs, which may change over time. A full reassessment is scheduled every six months for older adults in both the community program and the board and care project. However, if a client's mental or physical condition has changed significantly, a new assessment and problem update can be done more often.

(7) *Education:* Keeping clients as well as the vendors, staff, and board and care operators aware of current information and resources available to them is a vital function of case managers. Too often those who provide residential care are not aware of programs that could assist their residents.

(8) *Advocacy:* The case manager has a fundamental role to play in actively promoting quality care for board and care residents. For example, at every opportunity, residents should be made aware—as much as possible, given their individual abilities to comprehend—of their legal and medical rights. Residents must also know that their rights are not being violated by the board and care manager, the staff, or other residents, and that the case manager is someone who can be trusted to fight for the well-being and dignity of each and every person in the facility. Furthermore, case managers should emphasize to board and care operators and to federal, state, and local agencies the variety of services needed by clients. The case manager's advocacy role is particularly important when elders are unable or reluctant to articulate their own needs—especially where a State Ombudsman is unavailable.

(9) *Tracking the Cost of Service:* The case manager works within a budget when purchasing services for MSSP/CCFE, clients. Some clients may have special reasons for needing a lot of purchased services. It is the case manager's responsibility to track the cost of referred and purchased services, to monitor them, and to make adjustments when necessary.

(10) *Termination of Services:* Clients are terminated from MSSP/CCFE when they

- die;

- are in a skilled nursing facility (SNF) or intermediate care facility (ICF);

- are no longer certifiable for either an SNF or an ICF;

- lose their MediCal/Medicaid elegibility;

- request termination;

- move outside the City of Oakland or leave the CCFE project.

If a client feels that the termination was unfair, he or she may file a formal appeal. The case manager may be able to refer the client to another MSSP or CCFE site in another location or help the client get reinstated.

TWO SAMPLE CASES

Mr. G.

Mr. G. is a sixty-five-year-old cantankerous, suspicious, Hispanic male who lives in a board and care in Oakland. He walks with a noticeable limp and rarely smiles. He has no family and receives most of his emotional support from the facility's staff. He seems to be a loner. His medical records indicate a number of health problems: dementia (which significantly diminishes his mental capacity and reduces overall social abilities), a heart condition, psoriasis, and prostate problems compounded by a urinary dribble. He has already had one heart attack.

At present Mr. G.'s gait is unsteady. Transportation and a limited amount of socializing are provided by board and care staff who, in addition, pay close attention to the medications he takes and schedule his follow-up appointments with a physician, a podiatrist, and a dentist. The former two health-care professionals come to the facility as needed, while the board and care provides transportation to and from the dentist.

The case manager has identified several immediate needs:

(1) Mr. G. requires additional personal care assistance: his clothes are dirty; he has flakes on his shoulders; the skin on his hands is dry and scaly; and he has long, dirty fingernails. The CCFE project will purchase additional personal care services.

(2) He needs continual medical, dental, and podiatry treatment and follow-up to maximize his capacity to function at the board and

care level. These service needs will be filled by referred vendors who take Medicaid/MediCal and Medicare payments.

(3) Mr. G. continues to need protective undergarments and related items that will allow him to manage his urinary dribble. Again, a referral will be made to a MediCal/Medicaid/Medicare vendor. Having observed that Mr. G. finds it increasingly more difficult both to rise from a seated position and walk, the case manager will ask his primary medical doctor to write a MediCal treatment authorization request so that Mr. G. can be evaluated for a pair of lift shoes, a cane, and a seat lift to help him get to his feet more easily.

(4) Mr. G. continues to need the protective, supportive environment provided by the board and care. He trusts the case manager and states that he is satisfied in his present living arrangement.

Mrs. P.

This ninety-year-old African-American female is short and obese but friendly and talkative, though moderately confused. She has lived in a board and care for the past ten years. Her only informal support is provided by a seventy-two-year-old daughter and a son-in-law. Mrs. P. contends with multiple health problems, and her unmet need for an adjustable walker restricts her movements.

Mrs. P.'s health problems include impaired vision and poor hearing, arthritis, anemia, cardiovascular disease, hypertension, periods of mental confusion, and urinary incontinence. Her gait is unsteady even with the walker, which appears to be the wrong size. Members of the staff assist her with bathing, dressing, grooming, going to the doctor, managing her money, and using the telephone. Mrs. P. has started to see a new physician, and the board and care not only provides transportation but sees that an escort accompanies her. She is also visited by the house podiatrist every three months.

The case manager has identified several of Mrs. P.'s needs:

(1) Mrs. P. will require additional personal care assistance beyond that which is currently provided by the board and care if she is to manage her incontinence and remain in the facility. She needs to be escorted to the bathroom and placed on a bladder-control regimen.

(2) She currently receives and continues to need frequent and regular medical follow-ups, as well as podiatry care. Mrs. P.'s dentures are stained and do not appear to fit very well. This impairs her ability to speak clearly. The case manager will advise that she have a dental check, and will help the staff find a suitable dentist who will take Medicare/Medicaid patients.

(3) Mrs. P. needs to continue living in a supportive, protective environment where the staff realizes that she has periods of lucidity but many more days when she is very confused and vulnerable.

(4) She needs incontinency supplies but has refused to put on the type of disposable undergarments worn by most of the other residents with similar problems. The case manager will try to convince Mrs. P. to accept the protective underwear.

(5) Mrs. P. is talkative and quite sociable. The case manager will follow up on her need for social interaction by arranging for visits from a Senior Companion* several times a month.

The care plans for both Mr. G. and Mrs. P. will change as needed to reflect their levels of physical functioning and their mental status. In such situations, what are the case manager's on-going responsibilities to these elders?

THE CASE MANAGER'S RESPONSIBILITIES

It is the responsibility of the case manager to see that services, which often come from several different sources, are delivered to the client as needed. Each service should be delivered as a result of a need identified in the client's care plan.

In addition, the case manager must review the care plan of each client and make changes when appropriate. For example, changes will probably have to be made in Mr. G.'s care plan when he returns to the board and care after having rehabilitation for hip surgery next month. If Mrs. P. continues to gain weight, ambulates poorly with her walker, and mis-

---

*In the Senior Companion program, trained, low-income seniors can work a set number of hours each week visiting elders who are shut in and unable to get around. The Senior Companion is assigned to visit one or more elders on a regular schedule, and is paid a small stipend for each hour of companionship, which is exempt from Social Security income restrictions.

manages her incontinence, her care plan will require some changes or revisions.

Equally important is the case manager's function of tracking the cost of services to clients. Neither clients in community care nor those in board and cares can incur service expenses that would, in the end, exceed the cost of placing them in a skilled care nursing home. Occasionally, a client's income will exceed the allowable rate for MSSP/CCFE eligibility. These services will be terminated because the client receives excess income from Supplemental Security Income overpayments, income from some legal settlement, a spouse's pension, or the like. The case manager needs to keep this in mind and remain alert to the possibility that the client is out of compliance with the California State guidelines.

THE IMPORTANCE OF CASE MANAGEMENT TO BOARD AND CARES

Why, then, is case management so important for board and care residents? There are at least two perspectives from which to answer this question: (1) the residents' well-being and (2) the owners' ability to continue operating the facility while providing an adequate level of services.

Taking the residents' well-being as our point of departure, a case manager can observe current levels of care and assess the specific needs this care is designed to fulfill. He or she can assess the changes in an elder's requirements for care and arrange for additional intervention as needed. The implementation and effectiveness of all services provided can be monitored, thus enhancing residents' total health and happiness—quality of life—and prolonging residents' enjoyment of the special benefits offered in the residential care setting. Viewed from the owners' standpoint, case managers can not only secure additional needed services for residents, but, due to their knowledge of available community resources for the aged, they can make arrangements for lower-cost or referred services that may fulfill existing licensing mandates. This will help owners to remain cost effective while improving their public record and good name in both the community at large and the health-care industry.

For these reasons, it is our belief that information about the nature and function of case management is important not only for current board and care residents and operators but for all persons who are looking for a cost-effective care alternative, either to serve their own needs or those of a loved one. In the long run, such case management more than pays for itself.

NOTE

1. L. Gura, "Case Management and the Nurse," *Geriatric Nursing* (November/December 1984):372-75.

RESOURCES

For an in-depth study of case management from different perspectives, see the Fall 1988 issue of *Generations*, which focuses on just this topic.

For an in-depth study of reimbursement and long-term care financing, see the Spring 1988 issue of *Generations,* which focuses on this vital concern.

3

Sensory Deprivation and Its Consequences

In this chapter we will examine what happens to elders whose sensory faculties—sight, hearing, smell, taste, and touch—go unused, and the resulting apathy and loss of ability to respond to the world around them as these senses deteriorate. We will discuss each sense individually and explore what can happen when the senses diminish over time or cease to function effectively. Then we will suggest ways in which even small board and cares can, with adequate planning, stimulate or exercise these senses.

Detailed instructions for each sensory function are offered immediately following its analysis: for example, activities to stimulate visual acuity will follow the explanation of why the sense of sight needs to be stimulated. The resources that readers can draw upon for help are gathered together at the end of this chapter and grouped according to each specific sense.

In subsequent chapters the discussion will move beyond the five senses to address the importance of fulfilling several basic needs: the need to stimulate the memory, the need to improve and expand communication skills, and the need to become aware of our contemplative (or what many call the spiritual) dimension.

SENSORY DEPRIVATION: WHAT IS IT AND HOW DOES IT AFFECT THE BEHAVIOR OF OLDER ADULTS?

Will an understanding of the meaning of sensory deprivation help health-care professionals to better serve and care for the elderly? We think it

59

will. All of us receive large quantities of information through sight, touch, taste, smell, and hearing: our five senses draw the stimuli from the immediate environment, and then our minds interpret the data received. These sensations help us form appropriate responses to other people and to objects in our world. We receive sensory information from our internal organs, our external organ (the skin), as well as from muscles and tendons, and by way of nerve impulses.

During the aging process, the sensory information we receive gradually decreases and our perception is sometimes distorted. The elderly, for example, have neither the muscle strength nor the endurance they possessed in their younger years; they cannot grip objects as firmly as they used to or run as fast or as far as they once could. It is a rare older adult who possesses anything like the strength and endurance he or she had as a young person of twenty. What can this mean from the perspective of sensory deprivation? A back injury may occur while trying to pick up a load that years ago would have been scooped up without a moment's hesitation. Elders risk other physical injury because they misjudge their ability to exercise or to engage in hard physical labor.* Many can injure themselves as a result of reduced sensory functioning—in many cases, this involves poor vision. A significant number of falls, both minor slips and serious spills, have been the result of misjudging the height of a step when going up or down stairs. Older adults who wear bifocals often find it hard to judge proportional height, depth, or distance. Some elderly people fail to smell escaping gas in a closed room and thereby run the risk of being asphyxiated or seriously hurt in an explosion. Then there are the elders who may put something in their mouth yet fail to recognize the taste of a potentially harmful substance; or those who may enjoy taking walks but because of impaired hearing are unmindful of on-coming vehicles. Still others may not realize that a pan is hot and, in picking it up, subject themselves to a nasty burn.

There are many internal and external forces affecting the lives of elderly people every day. Yet, as we age and our senses lose the keen edge they once had, these same forces can become dangerous obstacles to our well-being. Much like unused muscles or skills that are allowed to languish unattended, when we do not continue consciously to exercise our senses their ability to function effectively is undermined. It is easy to understand

---

*How often have we read in the local newspaper about older adults collapsing during or soon after heavy lifting in the house, prolonged periods of exhausting yard work, or shoveling snow in winter?

that if students of the piano fail to practice, they soon lose the ability to play well, if at all; or if a singer's vocal chords are not exercised, they will cease to produce the lovely sounds that a well-trained vocalist can make. In the same way, if elders do not actively exercise their five senses, these vital receptors of information about the world will cease to function properly. Just as one's heart muscle will weaken and become more susceptible to heart attack without proper exercise, a sensible diet, and a less stressful lifestyle, so also our senses will weaken without adequate exercise and stimulation.

Why, then, do we consider healthy, well-functioning senses so important? The elderly as well as the young depend on taste, touch, hearing, sight, and smell for vital data about the world they live in. With the loss of fresh information, they become more isolated, withdrawn, and eventually cease to function. As this process of deterioration continues, elders become less and less able to respond to stimuli of any kind. Inactive, uninvolved, and uninspired residents—so frequently seen in board and cares—are often a direct result of the failure to continue introducing fresh stimuli into their lives. Unlike those of us who are highly mobile and able to relate to the environment on many levels, most board and care residents must rely on others to supply the sensory input they so desperately need.

In what follows, we will examine the specific impact that the loss or reduction of sensory capability has on the elderly.

VISION LOSS

Reduction or loss of vision may result from a number of common causes: for the most part, physical deterioration or disease is the culprit, but it might also occur as a result of accidental injury or genetic defect. The National Institute on Aging reminds us that "poor eyesight is not inevitable with (old) age. Some physical changes occur during the normal aging process that can cause a gradual decline in vision, but most older people maintain good eyesight into their eighties and beyond."[1]

Today, efforts to detect the early onset of cataracts* and glaucoma† can rectify these eye diseases with treatment or surgery. Barring known or unforeseen complications, even though a person is advanced in age, the prospect of a few more years of sight as a result of surgery or other

---

*The clouding of the lens of the eye.
†Gradual increase in tension and hardening of the eyeball.

appropriate treatment is of considerable value. In most cases, the physician is the best judge of both the condition and the proposed treatment; but there are instances in which a doctor might say to otherwise healthy elders: "Well, you're so old it isn't worth spending the money for surgery now." The elderly and those who care about them should *never* accept the "you're-too-old-so-why-bother" attitude. Such an attitude often attacks an already fragile sense of self-worth and can hasten both physical and mental decline.

Vision, like the other senses, diminishes with advanced age. Some of the changes that occur involve color perception, night vision, and the pupil's reaction to light. Imagine our surprise when one board and care operator told us that she had dimmed the lights in her facility to help reduce operating costs! This is just what residents don't need! Maintaining adequate levels of lighting would not only help her residents see better but also decrease their risk of accidents. It certainly would not be any savings if the operator were sued because a resident fell in a hallway or stairwell as a result of inadequate lighting. Estimates from the United Kingdom and the United States suggest that 50 percent of those over sixty-five years of age have visual impairments that are serious enough to require eyeglasses while reading.[2] Certainly, good lighting is vital for all who are conscientious about preserving their eyesight, but most particularly for the welfare of older people.

Another easily made improvement is in the *type* of light chosen for specific areas. Flourescent bulbs, found in so many public places, are not really as good for the eyes. According to the National Institute on Aging's publication titled *Aging and Your Eyes,* "incandescent light bulbs [regular light bulbs one would find in any household lamp] are better than fluorescent lights for older eyes." Regular lighting is brighter and more directed than fluorescent tube-type lighting. At a time when there is much emphasis on saving energy through the use of fluorescent lights, we need to be reminded that they do not necessarily serve the needs of everyone—especially those who require brighter surroundings.

The Eye: Complaints, Diseases, and Disorders

The same publication also lists the following common eye complaints, their symptoms, and likely remedies[3]:

Eye Complaints

Presbyopia: the gradual decline in ability to focus on close objects or see small print . . . can be compensated for through the wearing of glasses or contact lenses.

Floaters: the tiny specks that float across the eye, often seen on the periphery of vision . . . normal flaking of particles of tissue. If a sudden change occurs, call your doctor.

Dry eyes occur when tear glands produce too few tears. A special eyedrop solution can be prescribed to relieve it.

Excessive tears may be a sign of increased sensitivity to light, wind, or temperature. Sunglasses can help, but it can be a sign of more serious problems and should be checked by an ophthalmologist.

Eye Diseases in the Elderly

Cataracts are cloudy or opaque areas [occurring] in part or [in] all of the transparent lens located inside the eye . . . [they] usually develop gradually . . . [and] can be surgically removed safely.

Glaucoma occurs when there is too much fluid pressure in the eye, causing internal eye damage and gradually destroying vision. . . . Early diagnosis and treatment can control it . . . with eyedrops, oral medication, laser treatment, and, in some cases, surgery is used.

Retinal Disorders

Senile macular degeneration's [seeing spots] first signs are blurring or distortion of vision.

Diabetic retinopathy, a possible complication of diabetes, occurs when the small blood vessels that nourish the eye fail to function properly.

Retinal detachment is a separation of the inner and outer layers of the retina.

ASSISTIVE AIDS FOR THE VISUALLY IMPAIRED

There are special aids available to help improve reduced vision: telescopic glasses, light-filtering lenses, magnifying glasses, and a variety of electronic devices.

One such electronic aid is called VISTA,[4] produced by Telesensory Systems, Inc., which enlarges images so that readers with severe vision impairment can decipher them. The sheet of written material is placed on a shelf in the machine, which projects the image that appears onto a screen that looks like a computer or television monitor. It works well even for persons with very limited vision. Although such a device may prove too costly for most individuals to purchase, group homes will find the investment worth making.

A new type of laser surgery for the treatment of a wide range of eye problems has been developed by VISX Incorporated[5] located in California, and is currently undergoing clinical trials at several hospitals equipped with sophisticated eye surgery facilities.

DAILY EYE EXERCISES

Several simple eye-strengthening exercises should be a fundamental part of each day's exercise period. Board and care residents—indeed, all elderly persons—should be encouraged to perform them at other times as well. These exercises will not cure eye diseases or improve existing vision problems but they will help strengthen eye muscles (thus slowing further degeneration), make residents more conscious of their eyes, encourage the elderly to seek regular examinations (at optometrists and/or opthalmologists), and prompt them to be more protective of these precious windows on the world.*

(1) Open your eyes as wide as possible while lifting your eyebrows as high as you can. Stretch your brows as much as you can. Count to four slowly and then relax.

(2) Close your eyes tightly, bringing the brows down in a firm and pronounced frown. Hold for a slow count of four.

While performing the following exercises, do not move your head—move just your eyes:

(3) Look up, moving your eyeballs up as far as you can, as if you are looking at your eyebrows. Hold for a count of four.

*Here, as in all our descriptions of exercises and activities, we employ the second person pronoun "you," to address the elderly directly. References to staff and activity leaders are clearly indicated.

(4) Move your eyeballs to the right as far as you can, as if looking at your right ear or something far to the right of your head. (Don't turn your head.) Hold for a count of four.

(5) Look down, moving your eyeballs downward as if attempting to locate something on your lap, but don't bend your head. Maintain this position for a count of four.

(6) Move your eyeballs to the left as far as possible, as if looking at your left ear or some object far to the left. Once again, hold this position for a count of four.

Residents will note that when performing the exercises outlined above their eyes are moving in a clockwise direction. Exercise leaders may want to reverse the movements with the next repetition, rotating the eyes from left to right (counterclockwise). It is a good idea to give eye muscles a daily workout, especially since the exercises we describe here can be done *anytime* and virtually *anywhere*. Regular exercise not only strengthens eye muscles but helps to release tension in the face as well.

Studies suggest that the lens of the eye may yellow with age and may filter out colors at the higher-velocity blue end of the light spectrum.[6] Thus an older person may not be able to discriminate between shades of blue, between blue and green, or between blue and violet. For example, a ninety-year-old person might not be able to see blue flowers in a bouquet, because the blue blends with the green leaves. Similarly, an older person's choice of clothing may appear mismatched: even though the colors look fine to the elder who chose them, younger eyes with a more discriminating sense of color experience the hues as clashing. The elderly can more easily distinguish colors toward the lower-velocity yellow, red, and orange end of the spectrum.

What implications do these studies have for board and care owners? For the sake of safety and pleasure, these facts about color perception should be seriously considered when redecorating rooms or when printing information to be read by older eyes. Choosing colors that older persons can easily distinguish and recognize will enhance their living environment and reduce obstacles that instill uncertainty, self-doubt, and confusion. If board and care owners/operators expect their residents to read the various printed materials distributed by the facility—daily menus, instructions, newsletters, safety regulations, and so on—then the ability of elderly residents to discriminate among colors should be given careful consideration. Also, if it is important to warn residents about dangerous places, then using reds, oranges, and yellows will be much more effective. If owners of facilities want the background in an area of the building to fade into a nonobtrusive wall or barrier, then pale blues and greens are ideal. For some readers, the idea that color ranges and combinations have an effect on perception may appear strange, but to board and care residents whose sensitivity to the color spectrum has altered, they can make a considerable difference in both safety and pleasure.

Full-length books recorded on cassette tapes give visually impaired persons the satisfaction and pleasure of reading. Three sources for such recordings are:

(1) the local public library;

(2) Books on Tape, an organization from which audio cassettes can be rented or purchased;

(3) the National Library Service for the Blind and Physically Handicapped (NLS) operated by the Library of Congress.[7]

Audio cassette players with lightweight earphones can be purchased at reasonable cost. (The equipment will cost more if the purchaser also desires a record function.) When buying equipment, first consider the quality of the sound. Listen when someone is talking: can "s" or "t" sounds at the end of words be clearly heard? Screen the equipment for background hiss: does it interfere with gaining an understanding of the material on the tape? Does the clarity of the words spoken stay the same at both high and low volume? Are the controls clearly labeled or self-explanatory, and logically organized? Is there a tone control? Is there an earphone jack?[8] A good, quality recorder with a tone control and earphones can also compensate for various types of hearing loss.

HEARING LOSS

Partial or complete hearing loss affects one out of every eleven people in the United States. About 30 percent of adults over the age of sixty-five and 40 percent of those over seventy-five experience some degree of diminished hearing.[9] This common affliction affects many aspects of life: impairing communication with other people and reducing the ability to avoid many dangers (such as oncoming traffic). "Together, hearing loss and aging present a double disadvantage," according to Dr. Teena Wax and Lorraine DiPierto in their paper published by the National Information Center on Deafness and the American Speech-Language-Hearing Association.[10] Older people who experience hearing loss must learn to overcome their fears and self-consciousness and develop the coping skills needed to function in society. Simultaneously, health-care workers and others who provide services to hearing-impaired elders should be aware of techniques that make communication more effective. Otherwise, frustration on both sides will only aggravate an already confused relationship. Knowledge of these communication techniques and developing a trained staff who work with hearing-impaired residents every day can reduce the level of stress for both residents and caretakers.

Causes of hearing loss in the older adult population include:

(1) infections of the outer, middle, or inner ear;

(2) exposure to noise, especially very loud noises over a long period of time (many work environments pose or have posed a danger);

(3) blood clots;

(4) hereditary conditions or congenital deafness;

(5) bone growths in the middle ear (*otosclerosis*);

(6) adverse reactions to drugs or medications;

(7) natural hearing loss as a result of normal physical deterioration (known as *presbycusis*, it accounts for a large percentage of hearing loss);

(8) physical injury: e.g., blows to the ear or skull fractures;

(9) an inability to absorb salt into the system (*Meniere's disease*), which causes dizziness, nausea, and ringing of the ears (*tinnitis*).[11]

The telltale signs of diminished capacity to hear include reports by listeners that speakers are mumbling, talking too softly, or talking too fast; complaints by family members and friends that the volume on radios and televisions is turned up too loud; experiencing difficulty understanding words when conversing on the telephone; straining to hear while in church, at the movies, or at a family or social gathering.[12] In addition to these signs, several variations should be mentioned:

(1) a history of ear infections;

(2) talking loudly;

(3) complaining that others cannot be heard or understood;

(4) confusing words that have similar sounds;

(5) intently watching speakers' faces.[13]

COMMUNICATING MORE EFFECTIVELY WITH THE HEARING-IMPAIRED ELDERLY

The Hearing Society for the Bay Area, Inc., in San Francisco, produces and distributes a brief flyer titled "Tips for Talking to the Hard of Hearing." Mr. Sarley's cartoons help us to keep important points in mind when speaking to those with hearing loss. It is important that all persons who work or visit hearing-impaired residents study and follow these suggestions.

Most people with good hearing forget that they have developed speech mannerisms that often make it significantly more difficult for the hearing impaired to understand them. Consider these few strategies for effective communication:

(1) Talk at a moderate rate. Fast or slurred speech can be picked up by some people but even the so-called normal hearing person can miss much of what is said.

(2) Don't drop your voice at the end of each sentence. This is such a common practice that most of us aren't even aware that we do it. When this occurs, those who are hard of hearing often miss half of what is said.

(3) Speak as clearly as possible; be especially careful to pronounce consonants* well.

(4) Change from one subject to another more slowly than you would in the presence of someone who is not hearing impaired. Make sure your listener realizes that you are changing the subject. Use a key word or phrase at the beginning of your change to indicate that you are speaking about a different topic.[15]

---

*Consonants are all letters of the alphabet other than the primary vowels: "a," "e," "i," "o," and "u."

TIPS FOR TALKING TO THE HARD OF HEARING

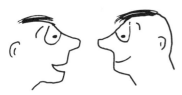

Face the hard of hearing person directly, and on the same level with him, whenever possible.

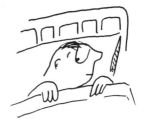

Recognize that hard of hearing people hear and understand less well when they are tired or ill.

If you are eating, chewing, smoking, etc., while talking, your speech will be more difficult to understand.

Keep your hands away from your face while talking.

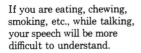

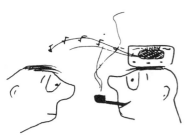

Reduce background noises when carrying on conversations — turn off the radio or TV.

Speak in a normal fashion without shouting. See that the light is not shining in the eyes of the hard of hearing person.

If a person has difficulty understanding something, find a different way of saying the same thing, rather than repeating the original words over and over.

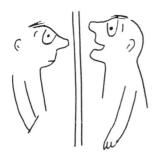

Never talk from another room. Be sure to get the person's attention before you start speaking to him.

HEARING SOCIETY *for the Bay Area, Inc.*

20 TENTH STREET   SAN FRANCISCO, CALIFORNIA 94103
(415) 863-4710 (Voice);   863-2550 (TDD)

A United Way Member Agency

PUBLICATION

Each of these suggestions reflects good manners and consideration for others. When people experience such sensory deprivation, the perceptual information received from the environment may not be clear enough to process. As a result, they respond in a way that seems unrelated to expected behavior. Then again, they might just walk away. Often the hearing impaired react in anger when they misunderstand others or are themselves misunderstood.

Keep in mind that it may be hard for the elderly to hear high-pitched sounds since this is one ability that deteriorates as advanced age approaches. (This fact bears a striking resemblance to our earlier discovery that older adults have difficulty perceiving color on the high-velocity end of the spectrum.) Speak clearly and at a normal speed but not in a loud or exaggerated manner: very loud voices will distort the sound of the message being conveyed. Try to speak clearly: mumbling is hard enough to decipher for those who have keen hearing, but next to impossible for persons suffering from partial or near complete hearing loss.

Another helpful practice is to face elderly people directly when speaking. As hearing loss increases, most people do develop some skills in lip reading. Again, this is something we don't often think about unless we experience some hearing loss ourselves or are associated with those who have difficulty hearing.

HOW CAREGIVERS CAN HELP ELDERS MANAGE THEIR HEARING LOSS

According to Drs. McFarland and Cox, the very act of suggesting that an elder consult a specialist is a crucial step toward helping the resident cope with hearing loss. They recommend that older adults who are suspected of having diminished hearing capacity "see an audiologist and an ear, nose, and throat (ENT) specialist." The audiologist can determine if the older person has a hearing loss and, if so, will isolate the type of loss and assess the degree to which the person's hearing is effected. The audiologist will run tests to discover the kind of hearing loss, the ability to understand speech, and the ability to discriminate between sounds. The ENT specialist will diagnose the presence of any medical problems and recommend treatment, which may include medication or surgery.[16] These professionals work as a team to help the hearing impaired.

HOW ELDERS WITH HEARING LOSS CAN IMPROVE THEIR HEARING OR COPE WITH THE LOSS

Wax and DiPietro remind us that hearing is a way of keeping in touch with the environment, of being alive and alert in the world. "Just hearing . . . the sound of children playing down the street helps a person feel 'connected' to what is happening all around us. The loss of this basic sense leaves some people with an empty, dull, or isolated feeling."[17] To relieve this problem, Wax and DiPietro offer various recommendations for elders who are trying to cope with hearing loss. The most difficult aspect of diminished hearing is what they call the social or symbolic level: "On this level we use our language to receive and understand language spoken to us. It means a loss of easy, relaxed, comfortable, ordinary, day-to-day conversation with family and friends." Wax and DiPietro continue:

> When you are not sure of what people are saying, you may become afraid of saying the wrong thing and thus appearing foolish, rude or inattentive. It's easy to lose confidence. The speaker, frustrated by your repeated misunderstanding, may talk less to you and may simplify and shorten spoken messages.
>
> Frustrated by your own failure to understand others, you may give up and withdraw psychologically, socially, and culturally. You may find yourself staying home or socializing with a few trusted companions instead of going to get-togethers, community events, or movies as you did before.[18]

In his book on deafness, Paul C. Higgins suggests several strategies that elders with hearing loss use to remain part of the larger community:

(1) pretending to understand, bluffing (nodding as if all is understood);

(2) being alert to situational cues that can substitute for the information missed; being alert to cues from other senses (the eyes); reading signs or brochures beforehand;

(3) making a prior agreement with a hearing companion to cover for them;

(4) accepting and acknowledging the hearing disability openly in social situations.[19]

One negative and unproductive strategy is to repress or deny the impairment altogether. Some elders with hearing problems may make excuses for themselves, saying, "I completely forgot," "I misplaced my hearing aid," or "I'm just tired."[20] For caregivers, being alert to these strategies of deception can help prevent conflict and hard feelings when interacting with hearing-impaired elders. The self-worth of these older adults should be continually reinforced by encouraging them to participate in group activities regardless of occasional embarrassing moments. Efforts should be made to teach board and care residents with better hearing how to be more patient and understanding toward those whose hearing has begun to fail. Upon witnessing derogatory statements about some hearing-impaired person, both caregivers and older adults whose hearing is intact should first take the speaker aside and explain the seemingly unusual behavior of the resident. If the statements persist, then it is appropriate to express a firm commitment to kindness which all residents are expected to honor. Such attempts to educate will improve attitudes toward hearing loss and make life better for all concerned.

AVAILABLE COMMUNICATION DEVICES FOR THE HEARING IMPAIRED

Older persons who experience varying levels of hearing loss are fortunate to have available a variety of assistive devices at their disposal. Some devices enhance the ability of elders to receive information, while in the case of those experiencing deafness, other devices serve as substitutes for the ability to hear. DiPietro, Williams, and Kaplan remind us that "persons with hearing impairments use such devices because they work and because they offer a means of being tuned in . . . to the larger society."[21] General categories of alerting devices or systems include:

(1) *flashing lights* that signal when someone is trying to communicate (e.g., a baby crying, a doorbell ringing, a telephone ringing, etc.);

(2) Dogs for the Deaf programs, based on the principle underlying seeing-eye dogs, train the animals to let hearing-impaired people know when the doorbell or the telephone rings, when someone is knocking at the door, etc.;

(3) a *wrist-worn vibrator* activated by a sound-sensitive transmitter in another room can alert a deaf person;

(4) *pagers* that signal through vibrating or by making a very loud sound;

(5) *telephone aids*: a specially wired receiver with a handset that allows the user to adjust the amplification;

(6) a *portable T-switch* slips over the telephone receiver but does not amplify the sound—instead it generates a magnetic field so that those with hearing aids can be alerted.

Telecommunication Devices for Deaf People (or TDDs) permit the hearing impaired to have telephone conversations via a print system. For example, deaf counselors may have such a set in their homes, through which clients with a compatible system can contact these professionals to receive their services. The caller's words appear as a printed message. When clients call, the counselors can call back and their response will also appear printed on the clients' receivers. Such TDDs have opened up a whole new world for the deaf and for those with severe hearing problems.*

In recent years, a great many television programs have appeared with "close captions" for deaf or hearing-impaired audiences. All three major television networks and many cable systems engage in close captioning, which allows the hearing impaired to enjoy art and entertainment and remain informed about local, national, and world events. Libraries throughout the country regularly show captioned films, and since most, if not all, new videotape releases are close captioned, the hearing impaired can join the hearing audience in enjoying a wide variety of programming. The hearing impaired could rent or buy programs from any number of retail commercial outlets or video supply catalogs, or borrow them from libraries.

Hearing aids are, of course, the most commonly used device among those who experience any level of hearing loss. Hearing aids are manufactured in a variety of styles and models; however, they must be properly fitted to meet the specific needs of the individual. A poor-fitting aid may go unused because it is too tight, too loose, or otherwise uncomfortable. Unfortunately, some types of hearing loss do not respond to any of the available models. For this reason persons who suspect that they are not hearing as well as they could or should are advised to consult a hearing specialist so that early diagnosis can detect the degree of hearing loss and possibly prevent further deterioration.

---

*Several of the resource groups at the end of this chapter provide their TDD numbers for the hearing impaired.

California's Department of Consumer Affairs offers these suggestions to individuals who may be contemplating the purchase of a hearing aid:

(1) Don't expect miracles. A hearing aid can only amplify sound—it can't restore lost hearing.

(2) Go to an established dealer, preferably one that your doctor has recommended. Don't patronize door-to-door salespeople or those who call you on the telephone saying that you have won a free hearing-aid test or some type of a gift. They will only add hidden costs to the price of your hearing device. Investigate the dealer by checking with the Better Business Bureau or with friends who may have purchased from the same dealer.

(3) Don't buy a hearing aid on the basis of appearance—a small one may not work for you. Don't let personal vanity cloud your judgment about such a purchase.

(4) Don't think that an expensive device is necessarily the best. The price tag is not always a barometer of quality.

(5) Don't borrow or lend a hearing aid—each one must be individually fitted to the intended wearer.[22]

While these are some of the tips offered to Californians by state employees who watch out for consumer interests, each state has its own agency to protect the rights of consumers. Local offices for consumer affairs can be found in most telephone directories.

ELDERS WITH HEARING LOSS CAN PARTICIPATE IN MOST ACTIVITIES

Older adults with hearing loss can participate in many facets of board and care life, provided activity leaders

(a) understand the cause(s) of the hearing loss and how to compensate for it,

(b) recognize the ways elders try to cope with their diminished hearing capacity,

(c) are able to follow the "tips for talking to the hard of hearing," which were discussed earlier.

Residents should be given clear, detailed, but easily understood instructions that permit ample time for those with hearing deficits to complete a given project or to join in the day's activity.

The fact that one or more residents can't hear very well should not be construed to mean that their joy, for example, in singing along to old familiar songs is any less real. Nor does it mean that they cannot participate in projects and activities of all kinds. *Being part of activities is the important thing.* Some older residents, like their younger counterparts, may never have been good singers or had always been told that they "couldn't carry a tune." But keep in mind that even those who are nearly deaf can *feel* the beat of instruments or the *rhythm* of music; they can, although in a somewhat limited way, join in the singing or just say the words. Alternatively, they can play a drum or shake a tambourine. Simple instructions can be found for making percussion instruments out of seed, small pebbles, and cans or boxes. The sharp sound of small pebbles in a decorated aluminum frozen juice can is audible to most people, except the totally deaf. Even those who are the most severely impaired can feel the "sound" of a piano chord or a drum beat via the vibrations that come through the floor or the furniture. Keeping in mind the difficulties those with hearing deficits have when sounds are high-pitched: volunteers or staff members who serve as accompanists for group songs should drop the key a bit lower than indicated on the score. As we age, it becomes easier to sing at a lower octave level.

Encourage all those with hearing loss to join in as many activities as possible. Don't belittle their efforts. Give praise lavishly. Laugh and enjoy yourself.

COMMUNICATION

Although there are no activities to strengthen the capacity to hear, to improve hearing acuity, or to repair hearing loss, we have offered suggestions to ease the conflict or frustration that can occur, both among and between hearing-impaired or deaf elders and the staff members who work with them. We believe that these suggestions will help eliminate barriers to communication between board and care residents and their caregivers. Good communication is important to the smooth functioning of residential care facilities. When residents don't hear well, they have a difficult time understanding the staff; they may convey inappropriate responses or refuse to respond at all. Because clear communication is so important, we want to do what we can to improve it.

Communication Disorders

The communication disorders that most frequently afflict older people are those affecting speech, language, and hearing. The problems associated with hearing loss have already been discussed. Now we would like to mention, briefly, other disorders that tend to hinder communication.

Aphasia

The inability to express oneself verbally is a complex problem that may, to varying degrees, reduce the person's ability to produce intelligible speech. In aphasia, the person has difficulty recognizing words, saying them, putting them in order, comprehending oral instructions, reading, or writing. Cardiovascular-cerebral stroke is the major cause of aphasia among older people.

Dysarthria

This condition interferes with the normal control of the speech mechanism, causing verbal expression to be slurred or otherwise difficult to understand. It results from an inability to produce speech sounds correctly; to maintain good breath control; and to coordinate the movements of lips, tongue, palate, and larynx. Dysarthria can be caused by stroke, accidents, and diseases such as Parkinsonism, multiple sclerosis, and bulbar palsy (paralysis of the motor sensors in the brain).

Voice Problems

The larynx or voice box actually produces one sound which lips and tongue form into speech. Cancer and other diseases cause nearly nine thousand patients a year to undergo larynectomy (surgical removal of the voice box). These patients, most of whom are elderly, can learn to speak again with voice prostheses or electronic devices.

Other Conditions

Brain diseases that result in progressive loss of mental faculties may affect memory; orientation to time, place, and people; and the organization of thought processes, all of which may result in reduced ability to communicate. An American Speech-Language-Hearing Association (ASHA) brochure explains the relationship between communication disorders and aging:

Our communication system which involves speaking, hearing and under-standing the speech of others, reading and writing, is a unique human development. It plays a vital role in all aspects of everyday life—our jobs, our families, our recreation. When communication processes are damaged by disorders of speech, language or hearing, the effects are always serious. . . . With the number of older adults growing rapidly and with the increased numbers of survivors of illnesses and accidents which can result in speech, language, and hearing disorders, more and more older adults with communications problems will be encountered.[23]

Tinnitus

Certainly the loss of hearing is a serious concern for older adults. But of equal importance to some elders is the common hearing ailment known as tinnitus, which often manifests itself as "ringing in the ears," though sufferers may experience buzzing, roaring, whistling, hissing, or high-pitched screeching. According to the American Tinnitus Association, "It can be a nerve-wracking condition which robs the sufferer of much of the joy and tranquility of life." The association contends that "12 million Americans suffer from tinnitus in its severe form and millions more have it to a lesser degree."[24] Since tinnitus is not considered a life-threatening disorder, there has not been much research on the causes of this often debilitating condition. We suspect that long-term allergies, ear infections from childhood, and perhaps certain medications may contribute to its severity.

The American Tinnitus Association suggests various self-help tech-niques that might alleviate the most annoying symptoms. These techniques will not stop the ringing noise but they may help tinnitus sufferers cope a bit better with the condition.

(1) Try to remain calm; use deep breathing or other relaxation tech-niques you may know.

(2) Simple exercises that require tension and release can help with relaxation, and they can be done anywhere: tense your shoulders, face, arms, hands, and any other muscle; hold the tension for a count of five; then relax as completely as possible.

(3) Use mental imagery to induce serenity: for example, bring to mind beautiful flowers, a peaceful scene, a favorite camping site, etc.

(4) Exercise every day: walk, swim, jog, play tennis or some other favorite sport. It will not only make you feel stronger but it provides

an opportunity to take out aggressions in a pleasant, productive way.

(5) Smile—happiness is catching.

(6) Try not to focus on the tinnitus; think of it as part of you, as something you have, like your hair color or your height.

(7) Learn as much as you can about the condition: remember, knowledge is power.

(8) Avoid loud noises as much as possible.

(9) Talk to others who share the condition, or join a tinnitus self-help group. Being in the company of understanding people is very helpful.

A list of tinnitus self-help groups can be obtained through the American Tinnitus Association (see the list of resources at the end of this chapter). If such a group does not exist in your area, then contact ATA about starting one of your own. Just think—you could be a catalyst for change in your community!

TASTE AND SMELL

Because it is so hard to conduct objective studies of the functions of taste and smell, very little is actually known about the physiological processes associated with the nature, development, and deterioration of these particular senses. Biomedical studies are fully documented: ear, nose, and throat specialists (ENTs) can diagnose and treat illnesses connected with the nose, mouth, tongue, and throat; but when it comes to explaining how the cells and nerves of the nose are associated with the ability to taste a flavor or recognize a particular smell and interpret its meaning (e.g., "smoke means fire, and fires are dangerous, so leave right away"), researchers are far less sure of themselves.

Much of the enjoyment of life is communicated through the senses of smell and taste (e.g., savory foods); smell and sight (fragrant and colorful roses); and smell, taste, and perception (e.g., recognizing a natural gas leak). We know that when our nasal passages (and the sinuses) are swollen shut by a cold or allergy, food just doesn't seem to have much taste. The flavor of the food is the same whether we can smell it or not, but certainly our enjoyment of that flavor will be significantly diminished.

Recent studies have shown that the ability to smell can be assessed fairly accurately by a "microencapsulated test of olfactory function"[25] in many people. Doty and his colleagues, who developed this test, found that the ability to identify odors reached a peak when test subjects were in their thirties, forties, and fifties; it decreased slightly when subjects reached their sixties and seventies, and decreased markedly when they were in their eighties. At all ages, women performed better on these olfactory tests than did men (probably because women have been sensitized to the idea that smelling good is very important to social acceptability).

Other researchers suggest that a decline in the ability to smell may be associated with age-related changes in the interior surfaces and nerves of the nose. Diseases of the nose and abuse of its lining and nerves— either by smoking or by breathing airborne pollutants—have a harmful effect on the nerves and cells of the respiratory system and therefore on the ability to smell. These contributing factors are also responsible for diminishing the sense of taste. One comment heard again and again from people who have chosen to give up tobacco is: "I can't believe how much better food tastes now that I've quit smoking!"

Certain systemic diseases, such as rheumatoid arthritis, can affect a person's ability to smell,* and a reduced capacity to smell may result from the side effects of medications prescribed to alleviate symptoms of various diseases. However, the loss of (or decreased ability to) smell affects the ability to taste, and since two-thirds of the taste sensation[26] depends on the ability to smell, this has serious implications for the nutrition levels of many elders, especially those who are in nursing homes or in board and care facilities. Research is being done to develop ways of compensating for a reduced or lost sense of taste and/or smell in order to heighten either or both.

Research into food identification has shown that the ability to perceive the odors of foods (odiferous gases given off by food) is particularly important to flavor perception (i.e., the belief that we are tasting something and the ability to recognize what it is).[27] Susan Schiffman is developing crystalline substances that can be sprinkled on food to stimulate or intensify their taste and color: "I am trying to enhance the flavor of foods so that old people will eat enough to get necessary vitamins and nutrients."[28] These flavor enhancers can have an encouraging effect on the nutrition of older adults: "We have to appeal to elderly people without making them feel old," says Schiffman.[29]

---

*as a result of the systematic swelling and inflammation of joints and associated tissues

COOKING AND BAKING TO STIMULATE TASTE AND SMELL

Most residents of board and care facilities have done at least some cooking in their years prior to entering the facility. If they have not actually prepared meals, they may have baked pastries or barbecued in the back yard or cooked over a campfire. Board and care staff members or volunteers should consider scheduling a regular baking and cooking hour each week.

Rolling out dough for cookies or pies, peeling vegetables for a salad or a main dish, stirring a pot of soup or a sauce are all activities that exercise the hands, arms, and eyes. The smell and taste of spices and flavorings delight the nose and taste buds. The texture of a crisp apple or cucumber on the tongue, the tartness or sweetness of fresh fruits, the tenderness of a custard or a ripe melon—these add interest and pleasure to daily life.

Once basic ingredients are mixed, the residents could knead a loaf of bread or roll out and cut pastries. Included in this valuable activity is the fun of sampling the results of their labors while building a sense of community with those who cooperate in the effort. Many a fascinating story has been told while participating elders were engaged in culinary enterprises.

Ethnic Food-fests

Special food-fests could be planned each month or as often as the residents and the staff desire. What a perfect time to encourage residents to participate in the preparations—especially in seasoning and tasting for proper flavor! If the board and care has residents of Hispanic background, a Mexican meal could be planned: soft, fresh, hot buttered tortillas might be a real hit. The elders could also make chili rellanos, tamales, and flan (a custard with caramelized base) for dessert.

Of course, residents need not stick with their own heritages for ideas. They could experiment with the cuisine of many cultures (Asian, European, African, South American) while they learn about good nutrition, gain knowledge of creative cooking techniques, try their hand at using new skills and kitchen tools, and enjoy the time spent in these creative group activities. Family members may want to help out by supplying many of the ingredients for these special meals, or serving as cooking instructors and/or servers for a particular ethnic or cultural style.

TOUCH

One sense that might not be thought of as a source of difficulty for the elderly is that of touch. Vicki Schmall, a gerontologist and assistant professor of family living in the School of Home Economics at Oregon State University, points out that

> studies suggest (there is) an age-related decline in the sensory system of touch. Skin sensitivity and the ability to detect pain decreases. It becomes more difficult for the person to distinguish textures and objects on the basis of touch alone . . . [the] pain threshold increases . . . [and the person is] less likely to perceive internal body pain or a rising temperature . . . [and] may result in an illness progressing to an advanced stage before detection.[30]

Some elders begin to notice that they cannot sense textures and surfaces—for example fabrics, wood, stone, their own skin or that of another person—as acutely as they once could when younger. The skin of these elderly persons, especially that of the hands, face, and feet, seems to have lost some of its sensitivity.* It is certainly true that the elasticity of the skin is reduced, causing wrinkles to develop.

Touching various shapes and textures, fabrics, furry animals, fuzzy leaves, or the soft skin of a baby are all pleasurable experiences. With reduced blood flow to the extremities (arms and hands, legs and feet), a warm pair of mittens or wool socks can feel very comforting. For the elder who experiences loss of vision, the effective use of touch can spell the difference between being mobile and being unable to get around. For example, braille floor markers on elevators can be very helpful. Maybe one day the use of soft chimes with universally discernible signals could indicate the specific floors in office and apartment buildings as well as on multi-floor residential care facilities. These are very helpful changes for individuals who suffer with the uncertainties of impaired vision. To enter an elevator and to be able to recognize the floor numbers in braille allows the nonsighted and those with extremely restricted vision to remain as independent as possible, no longer forced to wait for others to select the appropriate floor. And if voice or tonal signals indicate when a particular floor has been reached, this will add to the convenience level.

Some elderly persons do experience severe tenderness of the skin in

---

*This could be one of the contributing factors in the development of bed sores.

various parts of their bodies: they often find it hard to tolerate being touched. By and large, however, most people receive considerable comfort and pleasure from personal physical contact with others. Handshakes, hugs, and expressive gestures during conversation serve to validate the worth of elder residents and are received and returned with thoughtfulness and concern.

What about individual elders living in board and care facilities? Do staff caregivers have the time—do they take the time—to stroke a shoulder or arm, to gently press a hand, to touch a cheek or softly stroke a resident's hair? For most people, this kind of touch is comforting and brings pleasure. Soft stuffed animals are wonderful objects to touch, especially for elders who don't have a chance to stroke and caress live animals.

Dr. Schmall suggests that managers of board and cares should be careful about the temperature of bath water because elderly residents might scald themselves, especially since their skin is not as heat sensitive as it once was. Another danger, she warns, is that residents who suffer from diabetes may not sense a bruise or a cut, thereby paving the way for possible infections. These residents should be carefully monitored. Touch is important, then, not only for the many pleasurable sensations it brings to us but as a vehicle for noting dangerous situations as well.

The sense of touch can be stimulated in a number of ways including different kinds of sculpture, working with yarns, tying cords, gardening, preparing baked goods, and the exercise involved in handling equipment and tools. Board and care managers are encouraged to make arrangements with their local Humane Society to have someone visit with small petting animals. If the society has adequate staff to undertake a visit and specific animals trained to be taken to residential facilities, this could be one of the most popular events on the calendar. Be aware, however, that at some time in the past one or more residents may have had a frightening experience involving a particular type of animal; for them, such a visit could prove very agitating. In the same vein, there will be those residents who suffer from allergic reactions to fur or feathers. Caregivers staff should be knowledgeable of these potential problems and plan accordingly. (A quick survey of residents should elicit the needed information.) On the whole, however, such petting periods are received with much enthusiasm and thoroughly enjoyed by residents and staff members alike. The irresistible charm of pets often attracts even the most skeptical members of the group. A wide array of animals could be brought in for a visit: cats, dogs, rabbits, hamsters, guinea pigs, and even colorful bantam roosters.

CONCLUSION

Five well-honed senses are vital to everyone's quality of life. Those who have reached advanced age are no exception. At this point in life, however, more must be done on a conscious level to stimulate sensory capability. Measures must be taken to evaluate, monitor, and compensate for whatever degree of diminished sensory capacity elderly residents of board and cares might be experiencing. If a meaningful life of varied experiences is to be assured to our oldest citizens, then it is our collective responsibility—and by extention that of all board and cares—to increase and enhance, as best we can, the opportunities for sensory stimulation.

NOTES

1. National Institute on Aging, U.S. Department of Health and Human Services, "Age Page," *Aging and Your Eyes* (Washington, D.C.: National Institute of Health, 1987).

2. Vicki L. Schmall, *Growing Older: Sensory Changes.* PNW 196 (Corvallis, Ore.: Pacific Northwest Extension, March 1980).

3. National Institute on Aging, "Age Page."

4. VISTA, Telesensory Systems, Inc., 455 North Bernardo Avenue, P.O. Box 7455, Mountain View, CA 94039-0920.

5. VISX Incorporated, 919 Kifer Road, Sunnyvale, CA 94086.

6. Schmall, *Growing Older: Sensory Changes.*

7. Margaret Wylde, "Audio Cassette Books Compensate for Sensory Loss," *The Aging Connection* (April/May 1988).

8. Ibid.

9. Teena Wax (Rochester, N.Y.: National Technical Institute of the Deaf) and Lorraine DiPietro (National Information Center on Deafness, Gallaudet University, Washington, D.C., *Managing Hearing Loss in Later Life,* 1987).

10. Ibid.

11. Based on the Audiotone pamphlet #6617 Re, "The Sound Facts on Hearing," a Division of Lear Sigler, Inc., P.O. Box 2905, Phoenix, Ariz.; and William McFarland and B. Patricia Cox, *Aging and Hearing Loss: Some Commonly Asked Questions* (Washington, D.C.: National Information Service Center on Deafness, Gallaudet University, 1985).

12. Aural Rehabilitation Program (Hearing Reduction), Hearing Society for the Bay Area, Inc., 20-10th Street, #200, San Francisco, CA 94103.

13. McFarland and Cox, *Aging and Hearing Loss.*

14. Hearing Society for the Bay Area, Inc., "Tips for Talking to the Hard of Hearing."

15. Ibid.

16. McFarland and Cox, *Aging and Hearing Loss.*

17. Wax and DiPietro, *Managing Hearing Loss in Later Life.*

18. Ibid.

19. Paul C. Higgins, *Outsiders in a Hearing World: A Society of Deafness* (Beverly Hills, Calif.: Sage Publications, 1980).

20. Ibid.

21. American Speech-Language-Hearing Association *Communication Disorders and Aging,* by DiPietro, Williams, and Kaplan (Rockville, Md.: ASLHS, n.d.).

22. State of California Department of Consumer Affairs, 1020 N. Street, Sacramento, CA 95814 (1980).

23. Ibid.

24. American Tinnitus Association, *Tinnitus: Coping with Stress of Tinnitus* (Portland, Ore.: ATA, n.d.).

25. R. L. Doty, "Age-Related Changes in Smell," *American Family Physicians* (September 1985): 32C3, p. 221.

26. Schmall, *Growing Older: Sensory Changes.*

27. Murphy, "Age and Food Identification Ability," *Journal of Gerontology* 40 (1985): 47-52.

28. Susan Schiffman in Paul Berton's "New Tastes for Seniors," *Maclean's* 98 (December 1985).

29. Ibid.

30. Schmall, *Growing Older: Sensory Changes.*

RESOURCES*

Sight

American Academy of Ophthalmology
P.O. Box 7424
San Francisco, CA 94120-7424
(415) 561-8500

and

National Eye Care Project Helpline
P.O. Box 6988
San Francisco, CA 94120-6988
(800) 222-3973

---

*Some resources have been drawn from *The Resource Directory for Older People* published by the National Institute on Aging.

A professional society that gathers, studies, and publishes eye care information. Free publications available.

American Council of the Blind
Suite 1100
1010 Vermont Avenue NW
Washington, DC 20005
(202) 393-3666
Information Service
(800) 424-8666

Its purpose is to improve the living conditions of the blind and visually impaired. The council advocates for educational opportunities, health-care services, social security benefits, vocational training, and other health and social services.

American Foundation for the Blind
15 West 16th Street
New York, NY 10011
(212) 620-2147
(800) 232-5463 (information hotline)

Develops and provides programming and services to help the blind and visually impaired remain independent within the community. It distributes a *Directory of Services for Blind and Visually Impaired Persons in the United States* and provides a catalog of available publications. One such catalog is titled *Products for People with Vision Problems.* It describes products including clocks/timers/watches, games (e.g., braille Monopoly® and Scrabble®), calculators, communication devices, tools, instruments, kitchen and bath aids, and other health maintenance items.

American Optometric Association
243 North Lindbergh Boulevard
St. Louis, MO 63141
(314) 991-4100

This professional organization gathers, studies, and publishes eye-care information. It offers an Older Adult Screening Program that provides free vision screening through senior centers and community groups. Free publications are available.

Better Vision Institute
Suite 1310
1800 North Kent Street
Rosslyn, VA 22209
(703) 243-1528

This educational organization seeks to inform the public about the importance of vision care and regular eye examinations, as well as the prevention, detection, and treatment of eye diseases.

Bible Alliance, Inc.
P.O. Box 621
Bradenton, FL 34206

Provides free tapes of the Bible in several languages for the listening pleasure of those who are certified as legally blind.

Books on Tape
P.O. Box 7900
Newport Beach, CA 92658
(800) 626-3333
FAX (714) 548-6574

Audio cassettes can be rented or purchased. Rental prices range from $10.00 to over $20.00 per book, with $2.00 to $5.50 shipping and handling fee. Patrons may keep their selections for thirty days, with a modest penalty charge for overdue tapes. (Information provided by Margaret Wylde, Ph.D., Director of the Institute for Technology Development in Oxford, Mississippi. See note 7 above.)

Lions Blind Center and Outreach Services
3834 Opal Street
Oakland, CA 94609
(510) 654-2561

This is a national network that provides (1) educational/recreational classes; (2) workshop/rehabilitation programs for the visually impaired; (3) orientation and mobility specialists who work with developmentally disabled and visually impaired persons in their own homes as well as providing community-wide programming; and (4) assessment, instruction, and staff support for visually impaired clients in programs for those with developmental disabilities. Check your local telephone directory for the center nearest you.

National Association for the Visually Handicapped
22 West 21st Street
New York, NY 10011
(212) 889-3141

A voluntary health agency that works with the partially sighted.

National Eye Institute
Office of Scientific Reporting
Building 31, Room 6A29
Bethesda, MD 20892
(301) 496-5248

This institute helps to develop educational programs to prevent blindness and distributes public information brochures on such topics as cataracts, glaucoma, and diabetic retinopathy.

National Society to Prevent Blindness
500 East Remington Road
Schaumburg, IL 60173
(312) 843-2020
Information Service
(800) 221-3004

Publishes *Prevent Blindness News* three times each year, and provides pamphlets on eye safety, glaucoma, and eye examinations. The society also has an educational program for older adults called Lifesight: Growing Older with Good Vision.

Opticians Association of America
10341 Democracy Lane
P.O. Box 10110
Fairfax, VA 22030
(703) 691-8355

Will answer brief inquiries from the public about how to locate a licensed optician in your area.

Special Needs Catalog
Radio Shack
Department 88-A389
300 One Tandy Center
Fort Worth, TX 76102

Your local Radio Shack stores may also stock the catalog. Items in stock include: telephone aids, Digital Blood Pressure/Pulse Monitors, Vox (voice activated) players, door alarms, computers, and much more.

Talking Books Program

The National Library Service for the Blind and Physically Handicapped (NLS) is operated by the Library of Congress. The Talking Books Program provides special audiotapes and the systems needed to play them. Those seeking to qualify for the program can apply at any local library. (See Margaret Wylde at note 7 above.)

Vision Foundation
818 Mt. Auburn Street
Watertown, MA 02172

This foundation has published a free Vision Resource List that includes information on special products and services for the visually impaired.

VISTA
Telesensory Systems, Inc.
455 North Bernardo Avenue
P.O. Box 7455
Mountain View, CA 94039-0923

VISX Incorporated
919 Kifer Road
Sunnyvale, CA 94086

Hearing

American Speech-Language-Hearing Association (ASHA)
National Association for Hearing and Speech Action (NAHSA)
10801 Rockville Pike
Rockville, MD 20852
(301) 897-5700
Helpline
(800) 638-8255 (except Maryland)
(800) 638-9255 (TDD)
(301) 897-8682 (in Maryland)

Answers the public's questions about communication disorders and provides the names of certified audiologists to diagnose hearing problems and to fit individuals with hearing aids.

American Tinnitus Association
P.O. Box 5
Portland, OR 97207
(503) 248-9985

Voluntary organization that supports research to find a cure for tinnitus. It sponsors a nationwide network of self-help groups for tinnitus sufferers and their families. Offers referrals to service providers in the community.

Dizziness and Balance Disorders Association Resource Center
Room 300
1015 Northwest 22nd Avenue
Portland, OR 97210
(503) 229-7348

A nonprofit organization serving as a support network for those who are coping with dizziness and balance disorders. It may be of assistance to those who are experiencing hearing loss and associated problems.

Dogs for the Deaf
10175 Wheeler Road
Central Point, OR 97502
(503) 826-9220 (voice/TDD)

This organization provides deaf persons with Hearing Ear Dogs specially trained to direct their owners to such sounds as a door bell, telephone, smoke alarm, a baby's cry, or other designated sounds. According to the organization's pamphlet, the animals are rescued from pounds and shelters, trained, and delivered anywhere in the country to those who need them. There is no charge for the animal or the training. "Hearing Ear Dogs are allowed the same access rights to transportation, buildings, restaurants, markets, schools, and other public facilities as all guide dogs. Hearing Ear Dogs are easily identified by a blaze orange collar and leash; and the owner always carries a photo I.D."

Hearing Society for the Bay Area, Inc.
20-10th Street #200
San Francisco, CA 94103
(415) 863-4710

Provides information on resources available to those suffering form hearing loss. Individuals calling from outside the San Francisco area can be directed to those organizations and groups in their locality from whom help can be obtained.

National Association for the Deaf
814 Thayer Avenue
Silver Spring, MD 20910
(301) 587-1788 (voice and TDD)

This organization advocates on behalf of the deaf and disseminates information concerning deafness. It can provide a complete listing of organizations throughout the United States that provide services to deaf persons and their families.

National Information Center on Deafness (NICD)
Gallaudet University
800 Florida Avenue, NE
Washington, DC 20002
(202) 651-5051 (voice)
(202) 651-5052 (TDD)

Publishes useful informational pamphlets to help those with hearing loss or hearing difficulties.

National Institute on Deafness and Other Communication Disorders
Information Office
9000 Rockville Pike
Bethesda, MD 20892
(301) 496-5751

A national clearinghouse of information on diseases affecting hearing, balance, voice, speech, language, taste, and smell. A list of free publications is available.

Self-Help for Hard of Hearing People
7800 Wisconsin Avenue
Bethesda, MD 20814
(301) 657-2248 (voice)
(301) 657-2249 (TDD)

This nonprofit educational organization, concerned with the interests and welfare of the hearing impaired, provides support, encouragement, and information on detection and treatment of hearing loss. It also distributes relevant educational materials.

Additional

Check your local telephone directory to find information about available special services and assistive devices for sale or lease from the telephone company.

In Alameda County, California, the Naval Regional Medical facility (Oak Knoll Naval Hospital) 8750 Mountain Boulevard, Oakland, CA 94627 (510) 639-5268, provides audiology and speech pathology services for retired military persons and their dependents. Your local Veterans Administration Office should be able to tell you if such a facility is located in your area.

A call to your County Health Department or the County Department of Senior Services may prove worthwhile when seeking general information about or referral to organizations that serve the needs of a hearing impaired person.

Closed Captioning for the Hearing Impaired

Decoding machines can be hooked up to a television set. This device enables those with hearing disabilities to enjoy television programming and movies with the help of subtitles or captions. The decoder and all the necessary materials for installation can be purchased from:

Deaf Counseling, Advocacy and Referral Agency (DCARA)
157 Parrott Street
San Leandro, CA 94577
(510) 351-3937
(510) 351-3938

General Resources

Abramson, Marcia, and Paula M. Lovas, eds. *Aging and Sensory Change: An Annotated Bibliography* (Washington, D.C.: The Gerontology Society of America, 1988). This book not only presents the state-of-the-art synthesis of knowledge in this very important field, but indicates where research is needed. This bibliography, compiled by all disciplines relevant to the field of aging, inventories literature pertinent to an understanding of sensory deprivation. It is subdivided according to the respective senses.

Smell

Arlington, Richard. *Smelling.* Gig Harbor, Wash.: Raintree Publishers, 1985.
Berry, Joy A. *Teach Me about Smelling.* Danbury, Conn.: Grolier, Inc., 1986.
McPhee, Gribble. *Smells: Things to Do with Them.* New York: Penguin, 1978.
Van Toller, C., et al. *Aging and the Sense of Smell.* Springfield, Ill.: Charles C. Thomas, 1985.

Taste

Ache, B. W., et al., eds., *Perception of Complex Tastes and Smells.* San Diego, Calif.: Academic Press, 1988.
Allington, Richard L. *Tasting.* Gig Harbor, Wash.: Raintree Publishers, 1985.
Brillat-Savarin, Jean A. *The Physiology of Taste.* New Haven, Conn.: Leetes Island Books, 1982.
Moncure, Jane B. *A Tasting Party.* Chicago: Childrens Press, 1982.
Perry, Kate. *What's That Taste?* New York: Watts, Franklin, Inc., 1986.

Touch

Allington, Richard L. *Touching*. Gig Harbor, Wash.: Raintree Publishers, 1985.

Berry, Joy W. *Teach Me about Touching*. Danbury, Conn.: Grolier, Inc., 1986.

Colton, Helen. *The Gift of Touch: How Physical Contact Improves Communication, Pleasure, and Health*. New York: Putnam Publishing Group, 1983.

Moncure, Jane B. *The Touch Book*. Chicago: Childrens Press, 1982.

4

Memory Loss and Mental Health

One of the enduring social stereotypes of older people is that they are often forgetful or that their capacity for recalling information is significantly reduced. Yet, recent studies show that memory loss is not a "given"—it is not an inevitable component of old age. The cause(s) of diminished memory must be sought elsewhere. Actually, if memory functions are stimulated, not only is there no difference in ability to retain information but, because of their years of experiences, the memories of older people are much better— clearer and more well defined—than those of younger persons.

If we look at active, mentally alert people in their eighties and nineties, for the most part, they live—as most of us do—in environments that require continuous mental awareness. A great many elderly persons are involved in life—thinking, planning, anticipating new events, etc.—and they have other people in their lives. In other words, these elders regularly receive stimulating mental input. Rod Gibson's new book, *Your Memory, How to Keep It, How to Improve It,* points out that many of our human strengths and weaknesses may be related directly to our memory process:

> . . . memory makes us human—without it we could not experience love or hate, have families, build things, practice religion or even communicate with each other. Without memory, each man and woman would indeed be an island unto themselves. . . . [It] is the absolute keystone of the human learning experience.[1]

Compared to the environment and quality of life of the majority of our nation's elderly, most of whom live active and very full lives, the sterile

93

atmosphere in many board and cares shocks us with its depressing scene of deteriorating minds and bodies. It's certainly true that, much like the population at large, the vast majority of older adults are neither as active nor as productive as a few well-known members of their age group: e.g., the comedian George Burns, former Supreme Court Justice Thurgood Marshall, or the symphony conductor Leopold Stokowski, who signed a five-year recording contract at the age of ninety-five. However, as Gibson points out, we can continue to use our minds and our memories; or better still, we can never cease to use them and continue to have good working memories well into advanced old age.

"DIFFERENCES" THAT MAKE A DIFFERENCE

The vitality of famous symphony or choral conductors is quite amazing. If we want to look at examples of good memory retention, we need only examine their lives. What special something enables some of them to continue standing at the podium and conducting difficult major works well into their nineties? Their longevity is even more pronounced given the extraordinary mental demands of their work. Just take a look at a conductor's score: a single page can have a bar of notes for every instrument or voice part. The conductor must not only follow the score but interpret it: e.g., when to instruct the entire orchestra, or any part thereof, to play louder, softer, faster, slower, as well as when and how to blend the different tones, timbres, and colors of sound made by the various instruments. All the while, the conductor is sandwiched between the group of professional musicians in front of him and the audience at his back, each member of which has personal expectations for the evening's performance. The conductor is under extraordinary psychological pressure to bring out the very best in each performer and to capture the beauty of the score being played.

It's no wonder, then, that conductors live so long—*they love what they do!* Their enjoyment—the thrill of producing that special interpretation of a well-known classic—corresponds to the triggering of chemical reactions in the pleasure center of the brain.[2]

We marvel at the memory of one such as Arturo Toscanini, who conducted well into his nineties. Now, few are blessed with the strength of memory possessed by the Toscanini's of this world. In part this is because we do not share his genetic make-up, but it is also because we have not trained our minds from youth to achieve musical excellence as he has—frankly, most of us just don't have the mental capacity. But something that all of us can do is to continue to exercise our brains—read new books, explore new ideas, learn new skills—no matter what our age, extent of physical impairment, or level of intelligence. Gibson reminds us that "memory is a living process" by which he means that it can grow, develop, and be trained, or it can be destroyed by neglect and apathy.

How does this "living process" relate to our claim that elderly residents of board and cares can retain much of their sensory faculties and mental capabilities with the help of regular exercise and stimulation? If we look at the process by which memory retention can be enhanced through various techniques, and recognize different types of memory and how to make use of them, we may better understand why researchers claim that old age need not bring with it forgetfulness. In fact, being forgetful should be added to the scrap-heap of lingering stereotypes that have developed over the years: e.g., that old people are either crotchety and mean or dotingly sweet and helpful, that many elderly males are "dirty old men," that the elderly are not sexually interested or interesting let alone sexually active, that most older adults are doddering and can't remember where they are from one time to the next, and so on. So often these images rest upon one or at most a few encounters with older people and are then extended— without warrant or foundation—to the entire elderly population. Having said that the memory can be exercised, we need to appreciate the several types of memory we possess and use in our daily lives.

TYPES OF MEMORY

There are three types of memory: sensory memory, short-term memory, and long-term memory. *Sensory memories* are yielded within seconds of hearing, seeing, or smelling something. When, for example, the smell of natural gas in the house leads us to look for its source, our sensory memory triggers a deeper memory retained from experiences long since past—a linkage between the presence of the gas and the likelihood of an explosion or of asphyxiation.

Short-term memory is what we draw upon to look up a phone number, remember it long enough to dial a service, and, unless we are going to need it often, forget it soon thereafter. If the item we've just picked up is important to us, we may store it away in our memory, but if it's just a one-time telephone call, we won't retain it in our conscious memory.

Long-term memory is the most intriguing or mysterious of the three types because it is so little understood at present. How do we decide what we want to remember? What makes us remember one thing and not another? Why will one person remember an event vividly for life while someone else may not remember the event at all? There are many unanswered questions about long-term memory.

To see how memory works we can look at the circumstances that make one memory of an event remain vivid in many minds. We can then devise ways, as Rod Gibson has, to associate an event, picture, or person with something that is important or very familiar to us, and then use this technique as a tool to stimulate our memory.

Many people remember distinctly what they were doing on November 22, 1963, when President John F. Kennedy was assassinated. They associate what they were doing with a shocking, frightening, and tragic event that united their personal history with that of the nation. Many older adults clearly remember significant events and people that made an impression (positive or negative) on them during their lives: these memories are intimately associated with some strong emotion—love, joy, fear, hate, heartbreak, etc. Gibson reminds us that "it seems natural that someone living a passive, lonely existence would tend to remember the past times of intensity (of emotion): love, power, ambition, fear," and that these memories are preferable to today's boring, routine, and monotonous environment. This may explain why so many elders light up when someone starts talking about what happened decades ago, but seem strangely forgetful about what happened one day last week—just one of seven days of endless routine in the same place.

THE ADVANTAGES OF A STIMULATED MEMORY

Why should the enhanced memory of board and care residents be important to the staff? Wouldn't a more lethargic, uninvolved group of residents be easier to handle? Mentally alert, high-functioning residents are better able to follow instructions, more likely to remember where they are supposed to be (say, at meal time, activity time, or preparing for an outing), more responsive to taking their medication in a timely manner, and more adept at toileting (if they are being trained to manage incontinence) and any number of behaviors that can make them easier to work with. Increased memory among the elderly reduces not only the workload but also the stress that comes from having to repeat the same instructions over and over, day in and day out. Some elderly residents use forgetfulness as one of many attention-getting strategies. Appearing not to remember things may well mean that the staff has to communicate more often with the resident to acquire relevant information, which is just what many older persons seek—especially those who are starving for human contact. As we can see, *in some instances forgetfulness is a plea for help.*

Mentally alert residents are safer residents. They are less likely to wander off, leaving a wash basin to fill up unnoticed until water begins to seep through to the floor below or emerge from under their door. Nor will alert elders go outside and leave their room unlocked at night. They will not be so apt to wander away from the facility only to be returned by the police or by someone who recognizes them. (The potential dangers to which diminished memory exposes "wanderers" are readily apparent.) Working with residents who exercise their memories regularly means that there will be fewer instances in which board and care staff members and loved ones find themselves combing the neighborhood for a "lost" resident. In addition to the obvious advantages for caregivers, the benefits residents gain from a sharper memory can be measured in improved physical health, happiness (pleasure in day-to-day living), and an improved quality of life.

JOGGING THE MEMORY AND KEEPING IT ACTIVE

"Mnemonics is the art of improving or developing the memory," according to the *American Family and School Dictionary,*[3] and includes improving the ability for exercising short-term recall functions. Short-term memory can be defined as bringing to the fore fact, events, occurrences, dates, times of the very recent past such as earlier in the day, yesterday, last week or last month. Long-term memory tends to be more effective among elders, possibly because the specific incident or event was tied to something very important having high emotional impact, such as great fear, great joy, immense grief, or intense anger. It may have had a traumatic impact requiring a major change or disruption in the person's life or thinking, and memory of it can be triggered by some similar emotion. Perhaps a long-term memory may come to mind because a similar image or event arises. The elderly may see a picture of an event—for example, the 1906 San Francisco earthquake, or the recent Loma Prieta earthquake—which will bring back all the terrors they had felt as a child. These memories may spark recollections of details long since buried.

On the other hand, an elder with limited mobility and frail health, over a long period (perhaps years), would have weeks or months of sameness with little variation in daily routines and very little stimuli that would evoke strong emotions. It would be very easy indeed, to forget what happened yesterday or last week when there is a deadening sameness to each and every day. Strong emotional situations are now lacking or rare. Today's happenings are very much like yesterday's. Still, these short-term memory items are critical to the elder's present survival. So how, then, might we help elders train their short-term memory?

In their studies and work experience, the authors have found that encouraging elders to develop the simple habit of repeating an act regularly was helpful. For example, when unlocking the front (or back) door, set keys on the counter or table just inside the door or hang them on a hook positioned close by. Similarly, the very last thing done as one goes out the door is to take the keys off the hook (or table/counter) and unlock the door. A surprising amount of frustration and wasted time fumbling through pockets, purses, drawers, and the like can be avoided. Placing keys in the same spot each time one comes in or goes out the door is a logical and easy way to implement the habit. Other items could be similarly placed: e.g., a single location for an umbrella, eye-glasses, checkbook(s), bills to pay, and so on. This simple procedure can help reduce worry and frustration. This small bit of simple organization can keep our blood pressures lower and save us time and energy, not to mention anger.

Another method to jog short-term memory is to associate the item to be recalled with something that is very familiar that won't be forgotten. For example, remembering people's names when introduced can be both socially and professionally helpful. The trick is to acknowledge the person by repeating his or her name: "How do you do, Richard." Repeating his name during the conversation several times when appropriate will fix it in your mind. Let's say you have been introduced to Jim Carlson and you feel it is important to remember his name. How can you recall the name later? Was Jim an athletic looking man? A quick tie to "gym" could help with name recognition. Common names like Jim, John, Bill, and George are easy to forget unless they can be related to something that is easy to remember. Did he have red hair, particularly attractive eyes, or some other distinctive feature? Repeat his whole name. Say, "I'm pleased to meet you, Jim Carlson." Say his name to him in your conversation when appropriate.

Sometimes, if the need is to remember a word, it can be rhymed with another word or made into part of a chant containing several words. To remember a short shopping list, the most effective thing is to write it down. However, a memory list can be helpful if the written one is misplaced. Chances are that short lists will be remembered.

Write things down. Thank goodness for Post-its®, those small pads of colored paper with a sticky end that adheres to many surfaces. They are unobtrusive and so handy to use. When it's noticed that an item is getting low, for example the shampoo, write it down on a list in the bathroom. Don't wait till you get to the kitchen to write it down. Keep a note pad by the bedside. These handy pads allow elders to jot down the things they meant to do but forgot; now they can do them the next day. No one knows when something very important might need to be remembered. Chances are, it could be forgotten by morning. If the item or task is written down, then we have a better chance to get it done.

When going out to do errands, make a list of the things to be done. Develop it in logical sequence: for example, go to the bank to make a deposit, to the post office for stamps, to the department store to buy a gift, and the market for groceries. Start at the farthest point and work backward toward home. A note stuck to a purse or wallet with "bank," "post office," "shop," "store" written on it can save wear and tear on nerves, not to mention a more efficient use of time and transportation. Successful use of a list can create a good self-image: all the chores that needed doing got done in one trip.

The elderly should continue to exercise their minds: they should read, go to lectures or take classes, join advocacy groups and study the issues, learn new music or a different language, study major artists, take up painting. All of us should stretch our minds—reach beyond the usual to something different or more difficult. It enhances self-esteem when we succeed. Even if few of us become expert at a particular field, unless that was the aim to begin with, the very act of making the effort proves that we are able to try new things and do things we may have wanted to do when younger but didn't have time. Now we have time. It is crucial to continue to exercise our minds.

In an article titled "Memories Are Made of This," Sandra Blakeslee commented on the importance of good physical health to good memory functioning.[4] This seems perfectly logical but it isn't one we generally associate with memory training. It stands to reason that a healthy brain will function better. Regular exercise (fast walking, for example), especially out of doors, sends blood circulating through the system and up to the brain. Ms. Blakeslee notes, "a healthy heart is a key to a healthy memory." She also suggests that we check to see if there were any major changes in our lives, such as making a move; a death in the family or the loss of long-time, dear friends; children leaving home; or other emotion-laden events that could lead to chemical changes in the brain.

Earlier, we mentioned endorphins, chemicals the brain secretes when we do something we really enjoy. These chemicals affect our overall physical and mental well-being. Each of the above tips toward improving our memory functions can help improve our ability to remember, and that, in turn, gives us a sense of accomplishment, no matter how small, which is beneficial to our health.

For residents of facilities where routines make work easier for staff, who are busy just doing daily tasks, the temptation is very strong for staff to routinize the day for the elders. It certainly lets staff members function better, that is, get the essential daily chores done in a timely fashion. On the other hand, this kind of embedded routine can make life exceedingly dull for the residents. It is essential that various types of stimulating activities be offered each day to prevent the kind of mental atrophy that may make it easier for staff to get their job done. In the long run, mentally alert residents will make the work easier. It should also make the work more enjoyable, since residents will be active participants in the day's chores, not dull recipients of care. It is easier to work with people who remember to take their pills, or ready themselves for a meal, or follow instructions without endless repetitive directions. Unresponsiveness among residents affects the attitude of staff toward their care, thus making the dehumanizing of elders almost a natural reaction. From every point of view, a good functioning memory is good for both the elders and the professionals who work with them.

Memories are brought forth by strong emotional feelings, special events in life, repetition, and the associations in the mind that are triggered by any of these. The elderly are frequently the subject of social stereotyping that casts them as eccentric or forgetful. These harmful attitudes are all too often accepted by older adults as true, which deflates their self-image and numbs their feelings along with the memories projecting from them. These stereotypes may well have been based upon studies that pit the memory capacity of young psychology graduate students against the memory capacity of retired lay people who not only don't understand the general purpose of the tests but have different experiences and levels of education. No wonder older people don't do as well on these memory assessments as the young do!

Consider for a moment very active people in their eighties and nineties or even older, and think about how their environments affected their lives; then compare these experiences with the living conditions in board and care facilities that don't provide residents with stimulating mental as well as physical exercises. The contrast is very clear. It is understandable why so much value is placed on memory aids. If throughout our lives we had been surrounded by stimulating and exciting events, people, and activities, most probably we wouldn't need any prompting to bring relevant memories to mind. But most of us have not been so fortunate, because we didn't realize the importance of these things, or didn't have opportunities for these continuing experiences. Nevertheless, we can begin right now to stimulate our minds. "With training and practice . . . memory can actually be substantially improved at any age," says Robin West, who writes in the area of memory enhancement.[5]

The remainder of this chapter will describe opportunities for activities leaders, board and care staff members, or willing volunteers to organize, develop, structure, and conduct sessions that can help residents improve their mental well-being. These activities are primarily designed to strengthen the mental functions in general and those of the memory in particular. Other activities, listed separately and discussed in subsequent, chapters—such as crafts, music, spiritual study, humor, gardening, etc.— can also work to stimulate thinking and its application to activities beyond just the mind exercises we will describe here.

ACTIVITIES

Since many elders have mild to moderate cognitive impairment, it is important to rejuvenate their minds through mental exercises designed to improve memory functions, while at the same time continuing to stimulate their senses of sight and touch. Persons who have lived alone for long periods of time do not talk much; their vocal cords could be weakened. Finding it difficult to talk, they tend to avoid situations in which speaking is essential. For this reason, our first activity involves group discussion.

Introduction to Group Discussion

Leaders of a group discussion should try to select topics that are of interest to as many residents as possible. An interested group member is more likely to participate. Listen to what residents choose to focus upon when talking among themselves. Gaining knowledge about their respective backgrounds—e.g., their nationalities, ethnic/cultural heritage, the states in which they grew up, the types of neighborhoods they came from; the kind of work they did before retiring; special interests, hobbies, talents, etc.—should make early topic selection easy. Focusing on food/meals or health-care delivery often inspires an enthusiastic response.

Such group meetings should be scheduled regularly with a definite date, time, and topic announced. Resident participation is more likely under these circumstances than when the specifics of the meeting remain indefinite until the last minute. It might be helpful to schedule regular hours on two different days: one for a reminiscing-type discussion and one for discussing the news and events of the day. The news program can be based on articles in the daily paper or timed to follow the evening news.

Some residents may not have participated in this kind of discussion for a long time, and for others it could be their very first time. Don't watch the clock. Patience and persistence will bring benefits. When a general air of disinterest or reluctance to continue the discussion is sensed, it is time to bring the session to a graceful conclusion. Even if such discussions don't catch on right away, we recommend that staff hold the discussion hours. Gradually, residents will become accustomed to their availability, and group discussion sessions may well become one of the highlights of the week.

Topics for Discussion

Show and Tell

This time-honored approach has been successfully used in school settings for years. It is a good way to introduce residents to one another and the benefits of group discussion. Residents could bring

- photographs or pictures of early-model automobiles or family members;
- period clothing or furniture;
- beautiful quilts or afghans;
- souvenirs from significant events they may have attended (e.g., the World's Fair, the christening of a ship, traveling to another country or immigrating to the United States, etc.) or lived through (e.g., the Great Depression, the two world wars, fires, floods, etc.).

These are just some of the universal topics of interest that can be raised so that group members can share their thoughts. Often during these sessions the fond remembrances of some older adults will trigger long-forgotten memories of others, and the discussion is enriched by the perspectives of all who attend.

Home Town

A topic of continuing interest centers upon the various places that residents have called home over the years as well as the special features these elders are able to recall about them: the towns (both small and large) where they were born and/or went to school and what their education was like, their parents and relevant childhood experiences, their friends and what these special people are doing now, events and early memories. After permission has been obtained from the residents or their legal guardians and the facility's administrator, a review of residents' files* should contain some of this information, which will help discussion group leaders gather items that relate to the places and experiences of those interested in participating in the group: pictures, objects made in foreign lands or in specific parts of the United States, what various home towns or home states are famous for (if anything), and much more. The local library could render a valuable service here as well. In fact, a local librarian might be willing to speak to the group about certain historically significant items/ events. If finding some article related to a specific place of birth is difficult, try selecting items from the library that would be appropriate to the period. Pictures or books dealing with the years when many residents were growing up will stimulate their memories.

Family

Most people like to talk about their family: questions about family members often release a torrent of thoughts and feelings. Be prepared in case some of these emotions are negative or painful. It is unkind to stimulate a flood of emotions that you are not willing to cope with.

---

*Approval for a review of resident files could be difficult to obtain because of matters pertaining to confidentiality. Even if it were approved, such a review could be a very time-consuming process. It may prove just as helpful to have participants fill out a simple voluntary questionnaire concerning their place of birth, their childhood years, past employment, education, special interests, important events in their lives, etc. What a great mental exercise! It calls on the residents to organize their life histories and then answer questions!

Entertainment Classics

Songs and dances that were popular when many residents were children are part of the fond memories they love to relive and share. Current events, such as the death of a well-known politician, musician, stage or screen star could serve as the focal point for reminiscing about their glory days and appreciating their special talent (see below: "Death of a Famous Person").

News of the Day

Preparation for a discussion period based upon the *news of the day* could be made by reading the day's newspaper. Cut out pictures or articles that could be of interest or might have been mentioned in the day's news broadcasts. Vary the topics to be discussed. Don't just talk about the headlines. Read for items that could affect the residents directly (e.g., stories about Social Security, efforts to create a national health insurance system, catastrophic health insurance for the elderly, an age discrimination case, elder abuse, etc.). Share human interest stories (amazing rescues, reunions, or achievements), since they are particularly good for stimulating discussion.

These current events groups are significantly enhanced if visual aids can be provided: headlines about international issues such as the recent war in the Persian Gulf, the destruction of the Berlin Wall, or famine in Ethiopia are more fully appreciated if maps of the specific regions are available. In many vicinities enlarged maps of many areas of the world can be found in the public library or through travel agencies. If need be, the discussion leader could draw a rough map on large paper, using the newspaper or news magazine as a guide. Taping the map on the wall would give discussants a clear idea of where the incident or event took place, providing a geographic focus for the meeting. A call to local travel agencies or the automobile association may prove helpful in acquiring maps for such purposes. In other situations maps could be borrowed for a day or two; possibly the families of residents could help provide them.

Sports

Do not ignore sporting events. Professional sports are an interesting part of growing up in America. Many women as well as men may have been avid sports fans at one time. Maybe they still are. Bowling, tennis, and golf, as well as boxing, football, basketball, baseball, and hockey, are likely to be popular with older audiences.

It is important that these interests be maintained and encouraged. Group discussions can create an atmosphere that simulates going out to the stadium (court, arena, etc.) for a game. If enough interest exists, consider watching the World Series, the Super Bowl, the U.S. Open golf tournament, or any other major sporting event as one of the facility's special meetings. Have popcorn, sodas, coffee, or even hot dogs and hamburgers if the game is on the air close to mealtime. It will not hurt to break the regular meal schedule for special foods that residents remember eating when they went to the ballgame or when they took their children to various athletic events. Having the game brought into the living room is the next best thing to going to the stadium. Have a "tailgate party." Make it a fun time.

Death of a Famous Person: Reminders of Mortality

When a well-known person dies—for example, a movie star, a president, or a musician—residents are affected. They may feel connected to the famous person in some way, but in any case they are reminded of their own mortality. Birth and death are natural processes. Residents should be encouraged to share memories of the movies the celebrity starred in, play the songs of a renowned musician, or remember the many important deeds of the stateman. Discussion about death should be treated as a natural phenomenon, not as an occasion for fear. Talking about a death can reduce the dread of dying. Be careful not to dwell on the death in a morbid way (especially if the death was a suicide or a brutal murder). Be positive: share memories about the person, but do not avoid talking about death.

Intended Benefits

The residents who participate in discussion groups should achieve a growing awareness of events, objects, and people around them, not only in their immediate surroundings and the broader community nearest them but also in the world beyond. A greater interest in other people and enthusiasm for events help improve the general physical and mental health of most residents. Elenore Ashworth, author of the manual *Let's Talk,* offers the following observation:

> A reduction of apathy and general irritating behavior can come from stimulating discussions. Chronic boredom can increase the mental deterioration process of residents. Sensory stimulation is of great importance for those of the elderly who are in various degrees segregated from

the main stream of the community [as are residents of board and cares]. A lack of mental stimulation can mean the decline of one's ability to function.[6]

Ms. Ashworth suggests that each discussion session be structured to achieve maximum benefit for both residents and staff alike:

(1) Greet residents as they approach, touching their hand or arm, making sure that each is introduced to or knows the others.

(2) Use "bounce" questions to begin the session. Bounce questions are those which cannot be answered "yes" or "no" but require specific replies and should be framed in a humorous way that elicits laughter and creates a relaxed atmosphere. Select topics familiar to residents: for example, "How did you like the rolls you had for breakfast?" or "What made you decide to wear that shirt/dress today?"

(3) Introduce the day's topic for discussion. If a "show and tell" item was brought, have it prominently displayed.

(4) Use rewards (coffee, cookies, sweets) for participating, especially at first so that the event will become associated with something pleasurable.

(5) Thank each person for their participation. Remind them of the next time to gather for this purpose. Ending each discussion by having residents take the hand of the person next to them, or hugging each other, can build feelings of trust and caring among the participants.[7]

Maintaining an interest in what is happening in the world is important if residents are to remain alert and minimize boredom. Stimulating mental activities help maintain individual well-being. The brain, like any other part of the body, grows weak if not used: the expression "use it or lose it" certainly applies here. Discussing the news of the day, not just watching it on television, helps residents to maintain the ability to analyze events, to express ideas and feelings clearly and coherently, to recall past events or ideas, and to remain ever mindful that they are an important part of the world with something of value to contribute—not just passive, uninvolved observers.

Starting the Session

The following, adapted from Ashworth's manual, illustrates how a sample discussion session might be conducted:

(1) The discussion leader greets participants as they enter the room. Residents should be able to choose where to sit. The leader introduces residents who are new to the facility or who are not already known to the other participants. This is a good time for compliments: "What a lovely color your blouse (sweater, skirt, shirt, etc.) is!" or "How nice you look today." Chairs should be arranged in a circle so that all can see one another. It is important that each group member feels welcome and comfortable.

(2) Briefly point out the topic of discussion for the session and say: "We are interested in how you feel about (or what you remember about) this," or "Does this bring any memories to mind?" Encourage everyone to speak. Be aware that some people tend to monopolize the conversation, while others hold back. Call on the shy or quiet ones by name and solicit their participation with an inviting smile.

(3) Take the time to listen to those who speak slowly. If an impulsive or less patient person interrupts, the discussion can be put back on track with just a few words: "Wait Louise, let John finish his story, then you can share yours," or "Let's hear what John has to say first, then we can hear your story."

(4) Clues to potential topics can be derived from the informal conversations residents engage in. Make a note of these topics on three-by-five cards so that the interests of group members can be discussed. Or residents can be asked directly what types of topics they would like to discuss. Involve them in the decision-making process whenever and however possible. Make it *their* hour.

(5) Draw the discussion period to a close by saying something like, "Let's take a break for coffee" or "What a good place to stop for today." Thank everyone for participating and remind them of the next discussion hour and the topic on the agenda.

Possible Sources of Assistance for Discussion Groups

Board and care staff members may not always feel adequate to lead discussions on the news of the day or some other topic of special interest to residents. When this happens it might prove useful to ask a teacher from a local adult education facility or college to come and lead the group. Organizations for senior citizens (e.g., the AARP, the Gray Panthers, local senior centers or adult day-care facilities) or a nearby social or fraternal group (e.g., Rotary, Lions, Kiwanis, Elks, Moose, Chamber of Commerce, etc.) may have individuals on their speakers bureau who are willing to come and lead a group discussion on some specific topic. The group learns so much more if the leader is knowledgeable.

As we mentioned above, the use of maps and pictures helps give residents a chance to stretch their minds, to think about the causes and effects of incidents taking place in far-off lands.

Don't forget that the residents themselves represent a valuable resource. Former school teachers, librarians, doctors, nurses, lawyers, or professionals in the group may be willing to lead the discussion themselves. They may also be willing to do "homework" to focus the session.

NOTES

1. Rod Gibson, *Your Memory: How to Keep It, How to Improve It* (Boca Raton, Fla.: Globe Communications, 1990), pp. 2, 3.
2. Eileen Rockefeller Growald and Allan Luks, "Beyond Self: The Immunity of Samaritans," *American Health Magazine* (March 1988):51-53.
3. Random House, 1953.
4. *New Choices for the Best Years* 29, no. 11 (1989).
5. Robin West, *Mental Fitness Over 40* (Gainesville, Fla.: Triad Publishing Company, 1985).
6. Elenore Ashworth, *Let's Talk* (Berkeley, Calif.: L'Anciana Press, 1982).
7. Ibid.

RESOURCES

Books

Ashworth, Elenore E. *Let's Talk.* Berkeley, Calif : L'Anciana Press, 1982. This book grew out of Ms. Ashworth's experiences leading discussion groups at a retirement community. Based upon practical knowledge of what residents are actually capable of handling, *Let's Talk* covers a wide range of subjects that will help stimulate memory, thinking, speech, recall, and special interests. This volume can be of great help for those who want to lead challenging group sessions.

Bolles, Edmund Blair. *Remembering and Forgetting: Inquiries into the Nature of Memory.* New York: Walker and Company, 1988.

Gearing, B., M. Johnson, and T. Heller, eds. *Mental Health Problems in Old Age.* New York: John Wiley and Sons, 1988.

Gibson, Rod. *Your Memory: How to Keep It, How to Improve It.* Boca Raton, Fla.: Globe Communications Corp. (5401 N.W. Broken Sound Blvd., Boca Raton, FL 33487), 1990. This concise booklet gives solid information to the casual reader. The author's descriptions are brief but sufficient for board and care staff to understand and use. For more detailed study materials, check your local library for the works by Edmund Blair Bolles, Robin West, and Kenneth L. Higgbee.

Higbee, Kenneth L. *Your Memory: How It Works and How to Improve It.* New York: Simon & Schuster, 1988.

Sheridan, Carmel. *Failure Free Activities for the Alzheimer's Patient.* San Francisco: Cottage Books, 1987. This book was written expressly to help elders recall events or persons that affected them in their younger days. Although Ms. Sheridan's initial intent is to help the Alzheimer patient, the activities in her book would be helpful to all elders who may find their mental capacity has diminished.

———— *Memories Are Made of This.* San Francisco. Cottage Books, 1989. This work contains activities to help elders exercise their minds by stimulating the reminiscing functions: recalling, talking about past events, etc. Board and care staff members who have had no previous experience leading discussion groups will find it very helpful. Even discussion group veterans will appreciate having subjects/topics outlined in helpful, systematic ways.

West, Robin. *Memory Fitness Over 40.* Gainesville, Fla.: Triad Publishing Company, 1985.

Organizations

Cerebral Palsy Centers
The Cerebral Palsy Center for the Bay Area
4500 Lincoln Avenue
Oakland, CA 94602
(510) 531-3323

This organization provides work services, work adjustment services, and supportive rehabilitation services. The Adult Developmental Program includes services designed to increase independence and allow clients to move in the direction of the least restrictive environment that is both possible and safe for the elder. The areas stressed include: gross and fine motor skills, cognitive development, independent living, prevocational training, social development, physical therapy, exercise classes, basic education, horticulture, ceramics, drama, self-care skill learning, and individual and group counseling. Similar organizations may exist in your area.

Evergreen (program)
Catholic Charities
Department of Empowerment
797 Montague Street
San Leandro, CA 94577
(510) 895-2838

This is a day program for adults with developmental disabilities. Through program sessions they offer basic education, personal development, and creative leisure activities. Catholic Charities is active throughout the country. For more information contact your local diocese or Catholic Charities office for available programming in your area.

Memory Stimulation Aids

Sensory Stimulation Products for Alzheimer's-Type Dementia
and Geriatric Rehabilitation
5450 Barton Drive
Orlando, FL 32807
(800) 539-0390

This company's catalog offers products designed to help people with moderate to severe cognitive impairment. The products include games, puzzles, cassettes, etc., for persons with Alzheimer's-type dementia and for geriatric rehabilitation.

Additional Information

To obtain more information concerning resources directly available to you, contact your local Mental Health Department or County Office of Aging. They should be able to advise you on materials relevant to your needs. Don't be afraid to ask!

5

Spiritual Health

Although the spiritual and affective (emotion-related) aspects of human existence tend to be overlooked by a great many people, opinion polls conducted among elderly populations report that religion, or the spiritual aspect of life, not only continues to be a powerful influence but becomes increasingly more important with age. Many believe that by ignoring this side of themselves they risk being cut off from a whole portion of life, thus presenting only a two-dimensional—physical and mental—view of the human being. One unfortunate result of looking at the elderly in this narrowly focused way is that our efforts to bring dignity and enhanced quality to their lives are doomed at the outset because we fail to capture what they obviously see as their whole human essence and the deep-seated needs found within.

Questions about the role of humanity in the natural order and how human beings should relate to one another; about good and evil; and why we are here on earth (i.e., the purpose in life) are just a few of the penetrating concerns that have occupied the human community—the elderly included—throughout its history. These broad but compelling inquiries— what some call metaphysical, spiritual, or religious questions—have remained with us irrespective of whether we currently attend or did attend religious services or were brought up in households in which religion had little or no role to play. The importance of these concerns will vary from person to person and from time to time; for some they have virtually no significance, while for others they carry considerable weight. To ignore this aspect of our humanness because these more conceptual components of our being defy empirical proof or qualification in any scientific way is, in our opinion, to leave out an important aspect of life. Here again, we will find ourselves moving beyond the sensory to address a much overlooked component of human services.

Studies show that the elderly, more than any other age group, include a large number of devout believers, many of whom engage in personal devotions. David O. Moberg found during research for his book *Wholistic Christianity*[1] that 95 percent of those over the age of sixty-five pray, 45 percent say religious faith is an important influence in their lives, 49 percent attend church every week, yet 84 percent wish that their faith were even stronger. What does this say about residents of board and care homes?

We must not assume that all residents have the same religious background. If there are members of ethnic minority groups among them, then, in addition to Christianity and its variations there may well be Buddhists, followers of Islam, Jews, and nonbelievers. Even among Anglo-Europeans, it cannot be assumed that all are Christians. Board and care homes that list "religious preference" on their entrance questionnaires will be able to assess the needs of their residents. The question can be raised privately while investigating whether the prospective residents desire religious services on a regular weekly basis.

WEEKLY SERVICES

Board and care administrators can call churches in the nearby neighborhoods and ask the ministers if they would conduct services during the mid or late afternoon. It would make sense to start with residents who belong to churches in the immediate area of the home; the pastors of these churches would be logical first choices. If all parties are flexible, a workable schedule of weekly services can be arranged. Also, the clergy may be willing to contact their colleagues to develop a rotating schedule, thus reducing the load for any single minister.

Many churches now videotape and/or audiotape their Sunday services, which are then taken by volunteers to members who are sick or shut in and can't attend. If approached properly, these churches may agree to loan their videotapes. The tapes, along with a copy of the order of worship, would provide information on the hymns to be sung that day. Copies of the words can then be made available to residents so they can join in the singing.

When soliciting the services of clergy it must be made quite clear that proselytizing (pressure to join a particular church) or presenting a specific demoninational emphasis for the expressed purpose of recruiting members is neither desired nor permitted. Joining or not joining a church must always remain the free choice of the individual resident.

Both prospective visiting pastors and taped services from various churches should be screened to determine that what is stressed in weekly messages is the positive and loving aspect of spirituality. Those who stress the negative—e.g., "You're a sinner!" "We're all heading for the final Judgment and the wrath of God"—should be urged in the strongest possible terms to deemphasize God's wrath and focus on His love. The elderly need reassurance, consolation, and encouragement. They have enough obstacles to face without overpowering them with sin, guilt, and images of the "Final Judgment Day."

Residents who prefer not to attend services should never be forced, coaxed, or shamed into participating. Some residents want spiritual study or discussion but do not feel comfortable participating in a public worship service. Their preference should be respected. Likewise, there are many older people who have no religious preference at all, or who are agnostic, atheist, or just unconvinced. Their convictions warrant respect and tolerance. In fact, it might prove a lively source of debate if representative believers and nonbelievers came together to learn more about one another's point of view.

THE HUMAN NEED FOR THE SPIRITUAL

Since earliest recorded history, many human beings have looked to some kind of spiritual force to explain those things in their world that they could not otherwise understand: natural disasters, the passing of the seasons, and the meaning and purpose of human life and death, or others. The residents of board and care homes may enjoy studying and learning about Bible history, cultural folklore, or world religions from local clergy or seminary students. It is likely that various residents grew up going to church; one of them may therefore agree to lead a study group.

Collective Prayer

Shared prayers or meditations, where participants who so desire can give the name of a person upon whom they want everyone to focus their attention, help the group feel part of a caring community. Concern is expressed for someone they know who is ill or in need of help. Residents can ask that national leaders or people suffering from a disaster be uppermost in the group's mind. They can ask for support for themselves, their families, or others who are particularly dear to them, or someone they know who has experienced a painful loss.

Collective prayer or meditation helps lonely individuals feel less isolated. By focusing on someone else's need, people turn toward others instead of inward all the time. It also lets group members verbalize their hopes, fears, frustrations, and concerns. In turn, each person may come to more easily express feelings of loneliness, anger, loss, and anxiety, and to articulate special needs. These times are ideal for sharing personal joys, such as the engagement or marriage of a family member or friend, the birth of a grandchild or great-grandchild, or some other special accomplishment or honor. Sharing joys and problems brings elders closer together. Members of the group come to be viewed as belonging to a family. This is not a mere sentimental thought. In a very real way the board and care community is likely to be the family for its residents for the rest of their lives. It is important, therefore, to create a warm sense of being wanted, needed, loved, respected, and appreciated. Emotional and spiritual lives are strengthened, which will enhance the person's physical well-being.

RESOURCES FOR WORSHIP AND STUDY

Most public libraries have in their collections many books on religious traditions. Nearby clergy may be able to offer suggestions for those interested in obtaining more reading materials. In addition, many churches maintain their own private libraries, from which board and care staff might be able to borrow relevant materials. Some churches, temples, synagogues, or individual clergy donate used religious education materials that they no longer need. With a few well-placed inquiries, a board and care's interest in receiving such donations can be made known. Furthermore, the literature continues to expand: many books pertaining to adult religious instruction are published each year, and various denominations produce their own teaching tools. We describe below some of the most popular resources.

The Upper Room is a paperback devotional guide widely used in Protestant churches for daily meditations.[2] It is published monthly with a Scripture, a brief discussion, and daily prayers. This guide can be used on a weekly or periodic basis for regularly scheduled meditation. Those churches possessing extra copies of back issues might be willing to share them with residents. The activities director of the board and care, or an interested staff member or volunteer, could encourage one or more churches in the immediate vicinity to make a commitment to give enough copies of this publication to fill the needs of interested residents. Given the age of many older adults who currently reside in most board and cares, it is probable that a number of them attended services at some point in their lives, and may therefore find the daily study pages in the *Upper Room* enjoyable.

For those with impaired vision, resources for spiritual instruction now come in large print, on cassette tapes or records, and even on videotapes with audio voice-over. For the hearing impaired, close-captioned videotapes will allow maximum participation.

The Christian Bible is available in many languages. If there is no religious bookstore nearby, a letter to the wholesaler Cokesbury should be rewarded with information on where these religious materials can be found. (See the resource list at the end of this chapter.)

Telephone listings for various denominational headquarters (see your local Yellow Pages) can put board and cares and other residential care facilities in touch with available retired ministers in the vicinity. These clergy are often willing to hold study and worship services at the facility. Many seasoned parishioners from nearby churches also have experience leading Bible study classes and are willing to volunteer their help.

A healthy curiosity is always to be encouraged. Residents may wish to learn more about other faiths: Buddhism, Islam, Judaism, Hindi, Taoism, Shintoism, or the religious beliefs and practices of Native Americans. In reading books on these faiths, it is not unusual to find that the basic tenants of many major religions are quite similar; the Christian God may be called by many different names. Though the source of what is believed to be supernatural power may often be described differently, the basic content of the Old Testament Ten Commandments appears in dozens of faiths, as does the Golden Rule.

If no clergy or lay minister is available to lead a religious group or worship service, other guides or schedules for worship can be located at centers that supply religious books and information. A lexionary, or carefully planned weekly program of worship and study, lists Scripture selections and sermon ideas based upon specific passages of the Bible. The content of lexionaries has been developed by a committee of knowledgeable theologians from various seminaries; it follows a liturgical or church calendar year. *Preaching from the New Common Lexionary* by Craddock, Hayes, Holladay, and Tucker is a recent example.[3]

If the use of a formal, structured guide seems intimidating, and a retired minister or seminary student cannot be found, residents can select a book of the Bible, the Talmud, the Koran, or other religious (or secular but inspirational) work to study on their own. Local religious book stores may well have study guides to accompany this material; many such guides do exist.

Hymns are an important part of every worship service. Modern hymnals contain both old favorites and recently written inspirational songs. Hymns are usually grouped according to the church season (e.g., Christmas, Easter, Pentecost, etc.) or according to some specific inspirational purpose: giving praise, seeking mercy, giving thanks, or offering consolation. Sometimes churches have old hymnals to give away. Occasionally, publishing a request for materials in a denominational newspaper can bring results. Since older hymnals tend to be printed in very small type, many board and care residents may have a difficult time reading them. To correct this problem, local organizations for the blind frequently offer guidance in finding hymnals that contain larger print. Of course, the words of long-time favorite inspirational pieces could be printed by hand on lined paper. The use of broad felt-tip pens adds to the clarity of the letters and the words. Two or three verses per hymn are probably enough. These handmade hymnals could be stapled or spiral-bound for future use.

Developing a Relationship with a Church

One way to develop a working relationship with a nearby church is to contact its religious education department (or someone serving in that capacity) and arrange to have a representative meet the residents over dinner. Another possibility is to suggest that interested residents go to church school on Sunday morning and talk about their life experiences.* Young people are so familiar with the present and the recent past that they find it hard to believe that conditions could be so different from one generation to another (e.g., that people actually managed without television, relied on the radio for news and entertainment, or lived productive lives before the widespread use of the telephone or electricity). Also, many churches operate "Vacation Bible Schools" or urban day camps, which are often looking for volunteers to help lead classes and activities. Both the able elderly and youngsters will benefit greatly from this type of interaction.

Some churches will encourage their members to stop by the board and care to offer a ride to Sunday morning worship services. If a resident is going to share personal experiences with a class, arrangements could be made to have a parent of one of the children pick up the older adult that morning.

---

*Arrangements should be made with the pastor or Sunday School teacher well ahead of time.

Order of Worship

A worship program is commonly followed by churches throughout the country. (A sample service can be found in Appendix 6.) Though there may be numerous variations, a similar ordering of the service can be found in many denominations. Generally speaking, the words of the hymns are listed in the church bulletin or program by page numbers corresponding to the hymnal, as are responsive readings and Scripture references (because these books are usually available in the pew). Much of this information may be familiar to those who regularly attend Protestant worship services. For the unitiated it provides an idea of how services are structured.

Shorter services are also possible using hymns, Scripture, and prayers. In any case, the selection of hymns should be appropriate to the Scripture reading. As mentioned above, pertinent hymns can be located using the topical index found in the hymnal.

NOTES

1. David O. Moberg, "Spiritual Well-Being," in *Wholistic Christianity* by David O. Moberg (Elgin, Ill.: Brethren Press, 1985). See also, Geralyn Graf Magan and Evelyn L. Haught, *Well-Being and the Elderly: An Holistic View* (Washington, D.C.: American Association, 1986).

2. *The Upper Room,* published by The Upper Room, 1908 Grand Avenue, Nashville, TN 37202.

3. Fred B. Craddock, John H, Hayes, Carl R. Holladay, and Gene M. Tucker, *Preaching from the New Common Lexionary* (Nashville, Tenn.: Abingdon Press, 1985).

RESOURCES

In preparing this list of references, we have called upon the sources found in our own libraries. Obviously, activities coordinators will have at their disposal the breadth of materials available in their respective communities. Each denomination and faith has its own particular order of worship and specific liturgy; contact the church or temple closest to you for permission to use one or more of them. For example, the liturgy book of Buddhism contains many wonderfully wise statements that are excellent for a nondenominational study session. Buddhism is an ecclectic religion or way of life that appeals to many people who seek peace of mind in a hectic and stressful world.

Blair, Edward B. *Abingdon Bible Handbook*. Nashville, Tenn.: Abingdon Press, 1975. This volume was written to help the reader gain an intimate, personal understanding of the Bible. Unlike more conventional commentaries, this work includes historical background in its attempt to interpret the meaning of biblical passages.

Craddock, Fred B., John H. Hayes, Carl R. Hollaway, and Gene M. Tucker. *Preaching from the New Common Lexionary*. Nashville, Tenn.: Abingdon Press, 1985. Includes commentary.

Keller, Werner. *The Bible as History in Pictures*. New York: William Morrow & Co., 1968. This work contains 329 illustrations and 8 color plates through which Mr. Keller adds to our understanding of the places and events recorded in the Christian Bible.

McKinley, John. *Creative Methods for Adult Classes*. St. Louis, Mo.: Bethany Press, 1960.

Phillips, J. B. *The New Testament in Modern English*. London: Geoffrey Bles, 1960.

The Upper Room (Nashville, Tenn.: The Upper Room). Published monthly, this small paperback devotional guide contains a Scripture selection for each day of the month, a meditation that relates daily activity to the passage, and a short prayer. It can be used as the basis for daily meditation periods, regularly scheduled Bible study, or weekly worship sessions.

The Way: The Living Bible (illustrated) by the editors of *Campus Life Magazine*. Wheaton, Ill.: Tyndale House Publishers, 1980. A modern language translation of the Bible; very easy to read and understand.

Weavings: Woven Together in Love. Nashville, Tenn.: Christian Spiritual Life. This publication is a collection of inspirational essays written by various contributors and can serve as the basis for religious study periods.

Cokesbury, a religious materials wholesaler, is located at P.O. Box 801, Nashville, TN 37202.

This company publishes an annual catalog containing church curricula and helpful aids for facilitating worship and religious study.

The above materials are suggestions only: the specific books, readings, selections, and instruction will vary with the resident base of the board and care facility. Some elders who were raised in a predominantly conservative Christian environment may believe that religious beliefs different from their own are wrong. Attempts to introduce nontraditional religious views or even interdenominational perspectives will have to be approached very carefully. Equally important is the need to respect the rights of nonbelievers.

6

Art Therapy

Art enhances the sense of sight with the help of color, shapes, and lines; it stimulates the sense of touch with textures, sizes, and shapes. Bringing arts and crafts into the board and care setting can be very therapeutic because they focus one's entire attention on the work at hand and, for a while at least, frustration, concern, loneliness, and anxiety melt away as attention is directed toward the project. Crafts involving cutting and pasting can be as simple as developing collages of pictures cut from a retail catalog or as elaborate as a Japanese kataezome, in which colored paper of varying textures is glued to a background.

A wall-sized collage created from pictures cut out of old magazines can be used by residents to tell a story in a much more interesting way than a rambling, spoken account. But to engage in this activity effectively, residents need a rich supply of materials from which ideas can emerge and take shape. Women's groups, senior center participants, or other civic organizations can be contacted to donate a wide variety of magazines for use as sources of pictures. Friends and neighbors could save catalogs and colorful circulars; in so doing, they become part of the board and care's community involvement. Free publications, advertisements that come with the daily newspaper, or mail-order catalogs have colorful illustrations. Even nearby offices or businesses, such as doctors, dentists, lawyers, and manufacturers, would probably cooperate if asked, provided the materials were collected in a timely manner.

HOW TO START A CLASS

Inquiries directed to adult education departments at local high schools or community colleges will sometimes result in a teacher volunteer who will agree to meet with residents on a weekly basis and lead creative arts activities. Most schools require a minimum of fifteen participants before they will commit to sending a teacher. If the board and care is not large enough to draw the minimum number of interested residents, people from local groups or the surrounding community could be invited to join the class. A staff member of the residential care facility or a motivated family member can also lead this type of activity.

COLLAGES

Much can be done with paste or glue and a pair of scissors.* Cutting out fascinating images and arranging them on paper is a very expressive medium. Here are some basic ideas for interesting collages:

- a collection of items focusing on a single theme or subject—e.g., fruits, animals, colors, hair styles, plants, types of buildings or houses, types of cars, etc.;

- a travelogue showing locations, signs along the way, people one might meet, or places to see on the trip;

- a landscape showing flowers, trees, and shrubs (It could also be an imaginary location. What possibilities for a fanciful journey!);

- creating a map of the resident's home state, indicating items manufactured, grown, or provided by the particular region;

- a collection of different groups of people—different races, occupations, ages, nationalities, etc.;

- an arrangement of cheery colors.

---

*Take care that cutting utensils are safe for all residents to use. Many types of round-tipped scissors are available, some with large handles for those who may have arthritis or unsteady hands.

Residents can let their imaginations wander; there is no limit to the possibilities in collage art. Pictures can be combined with colors and embellished using felt-tip pens and paints, yarns, or anything on hand.

To protect completed artwork many people use lamination, a process by which a thin plastic coating is affixed to a flat surface to seal it from moisture, fading, and cracking. Most school districts have some type of laminating equipment; ask for permission to run residents' pictures through it. If this option isn't available, try using laminate plastic sheeting from a local art supply store. This material can assure the long life of a treasured creation, and all you need to seal it is a warm iron. Laminated collage placemats are easy to clean and reuse and can really dress up a table or tray, or they can be mounted as wall hangings.

The Uses of Collages

Collage art can be used to decorate boxes that store the board and care activities materials, shoe boxes that hold personal possessions, photo albums, and many other things. For residents with reasonably good manual dexterity, collage art can assist in the making of party favors—for holding nuts and candy—by using plastic cups decorated with paints, pasted pictures, and/or colorful yarns. Colorful placemats can highlight a birthday or other special occasion, and handmade greeting cards bring special joy to friends and loved ones.

Since collages are by definition collections of things, they have a common theme: a particular activity, a month of the year, one of the four seasons, a special color, an important event or occasion. In smaller groups, residents can capture their own feelings by finding colors, shapes, and expressive faces or action poses that convey how they feel about themselves and the world around them. A picture really can be worth a thousand words.

Equipment and Supplies

For this activity residents will need:

- scissors (blunt points for those who are less steady)
- nontoxic paste
- felt-tip colored pens

- rulers (preferably ones with rounded edges
- 11-by-15-inch poster paper on which the pictures will be mounted
- old magazines, catalogs, used greeting cards, newspapers, advertising flyers, etc.

Procedure

1. Have equipment and supplies assembled. Ample table space will be needed for the artists to work.

2. At the first few arts and crafts sessions, suggest topics for residents to consider, at least until they are ready to develop an idea of their own. Residents should be encouraged to depict whatever appeals to them: ideas can come from the pictures they see or from some past experience that has special meaning for them. Self-expression is the key!

3. Artists can cut out pictures and paste them either at random or in any appealing order. *There is no right or wrong way to proceed— that's the fun of it!*

4. Residents should be encouraged to share their collages with one another when the artworks are completed, and to discuss what they were attempting to make and how they went about doing it.

Intended Benefits

- Making collages exercises the fingers and the hands; sharpens the vision (thus enhancing hand-eye coordination); and stimulates mental discipline in the selection process—that is, choosing from among available items when constructing the collage.

- Discussion stimulates participants' memories and encourages them to share ideas and experiences. It helps to exercise vocal cords, tongue, mouth, and increases basic communication skills. Memories of events, people, or places from childhood (or any time in life) can be happy or sad. *It's all right to cry over a sad memory, and it's wonderful to laugh over a funny one. Both emotions can be therapeutic.*

- Collage art offers many reluctant artists an opportunity to begin developing their latent creativity, and to keep the senses of touch, sight, speech, and hearing at optimal working levels.

- Collages are fun and they don't require special skills or training. Nearly everyone can enjoy a level of success.

- The sharing that takes place during the activity of making collages helps the artists order their thinking and express their ideas. For some this will be their first attempt at public speaking. A supportive atmosphere is vital. A wonderful moment can happen as residents display and discuss their work: many will see an idea or image that no one else has and express it in their own unique way. *What an esteem-building experience!* The finished collage can spark all sorts of memories that trigger emotions in both the artist and the viewer, yet it is for the most part a totally random selection of images.

- Another delightful consequence of making collages is the unexpected picture that actually develops. The final outcome can be a fascinating surprise to everyone.

Each craft session should be limited to no more than an hour and a half. Let it be a time to anticipate, not a period that will tax residents' stamina.

A Variation: Kataezome

The same "cut and paste" activity can be employed to create charming and evocative silhouettes by pasting one paper image atop another. The contrasting colors as well as light and dark densities of hue accentuate the images created.

Along with making use of scissors and paste, print or catalog pictures are replaced by simple or complex forms traced on and cut from pieces of construction paper. The background could be as simple as blank newsprint paper, which can be obtained (with some luck) by asking your local news publishing plant for the leftover ends of newsprint rolls. The exercise is far more beneficial if traced forms are discouraged: emphasis should be placed on residents using their imaginations to create free-form images. Closing their eyes, residents can think of an attractive form that they then proceed to "carve" in paper with scissors. The charm of *Kataezome* lies in the spontaneity or unstructured nature of the images. For some, tracing will be preferable, but this should be to help define the form, not as a cut line.

Once the figure or shape is established and cut, residents can paste the segments onto a piece of blank construction paper. When the picture is complete the entire work is then be pasted on a larger piece of contrasting

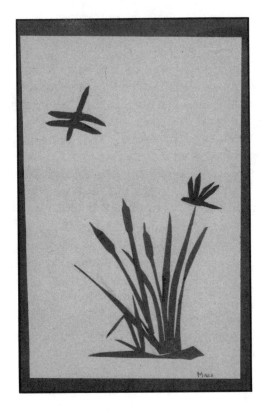

paper. In our sample, we cut brown cat tails and red dragonflies and pasted them on a light yellow background. The entire picture was then highlighted by being placed on a dark brown sheet of construction paper.

Artists can sign their names to these creations. A bulletin board display might be developed in a communal area of the facility, or residents could hang their artistic efforts in their rooms. Some board and care facilities sponsor art shows for families and friends.

WORKING WITH YARNS, STRING, AND CORDS

Decorative *yarn crafts* can be a source of great pleasure while at the same time helping to maintain residents' manual dexterity. Tying a simple yarn doll to hang on a door or pin to a shirt pocket is an activity that combines finger exercise with stimulating both sight and memory as participants associate certain colors with specific holidays, occasions, or events.

Macrame, or knot tying, emphasizes hand-eye coordination; and with each completed project residents will gain a sense of accomplishment. What was once an essential part of survival for sailors has been transformed into an art for creating useful and attractive items such as handbags, belts, or decorative wall hangings, all of which make wonderful gifts.

Afghans, hand-knitted or hooked blankets, can be made by those whose fingers are stiffened by arthritis, because the needles and stitches are very large and do not require intricate work. Smaller, lightweight afghans are wonderful for warming the legs, and larger ones can serve as attractive bedspreads. Residents who become adept at hooking afghans will be delighted at the new developments and beautiful designs available in this popular craft.

Afghan stitches are the easiest of all stitches. Pot holders, lap or bed robes, scarfs, and clothing of all types can be made using the afghan stitch, which is dense and like a cloth-weave. Board and care residents can get together and make a full, double-bed-sized afghan: many patterns begin by combining eight-to-ten-inch squares. For some this will bring back delightful memories of the old quilting bees. Instruction books show a remarkable variety of lovely patterns.

How to Make a Yarn Doll

Supplies

- A selection of colored 4-ply (or thicker) yarn will be needed. If only 2- or 3-ply yarns are available, double the length. (If nearby church groups know that the board and care wants their scraps of yarn, they probably will be happy to share them.) Select colors to fit a holiday: Halloween, Valentine's Day, Thanksgiving, Christmas, Fourth of July, etc.

- scissors (again, the blunt-end variety is suggested)

- a package of ¾-inch (or larger) safety pins (gold pins look nice)

Instructions

1. Select the color of yarn you like best. Those who are visually impaired find that bright colors—reds, greens, oranges, etc.—are easier to work with.

2. Cut the yarn into 4-foot lengths, for each person one piece each for a doll. Cut 12-inch lengths of yarn of the same or a contrasting color to tie the dolls.

3. Spread the fingers of one hand slightly, just enough so that the space between the extended index finger and the little finger is about 3 inches. With one end of the yarn positioned at the little finger, wrap one of the long pieces of yarn loosely around these fingers so that the body of the doll will be approximately 3 inches tall. When finished wrapping, both ends of the yarn should be at the bottom of your hand, near your little finger. Close the fingers of your hand and remove the rolled yarn.

4. Move to the end of the rolled yarn opposite the loose, dangling pieces and, using one of the small pieces of yarn, tie it off about one-half-inch in from the end. This will form the doll's head. Pull the tying yarn tight using a square knot; let it hang or tie it in a bow. (Assistance may be needed at first for those participants who do not have much strength in their hands.)

5. Now go to the bottom of the doll and cut this dangling end to form a skirt, or divide the cut ends and tie them to make legs. To give the doll more form, tie 3 strands on both sides to create arms and hands.

6. A safety pin can then be fastened to the "back," to make a decorative fashion accessory, or a length of yarn could be run through its "head" to create a beautiful hanging ornament or conversation piece. If residents are able and interested, they can stitch tiny facial features on the head. The charm of this doll lies in its simplicity. It merely suggests a human figure, as many dolls do, and does not really need decoration, though special accents are fun and add distinction.

At Christmas time residents could create colorful hand dolls to hang on the facility's tree. If each resident has his or her own tree, the dolls can be used to decorate individual rooms. For each mini-tree, cut two juniper branches and tie them back to back on the flat side; then stand them in a bottle of water. (Be careful that the bottle doesn't tip over!) These trees can be decorated with dolls that have glitter or sequins on them, or dolls created from silver or gold yarn for that festive seasonal look.

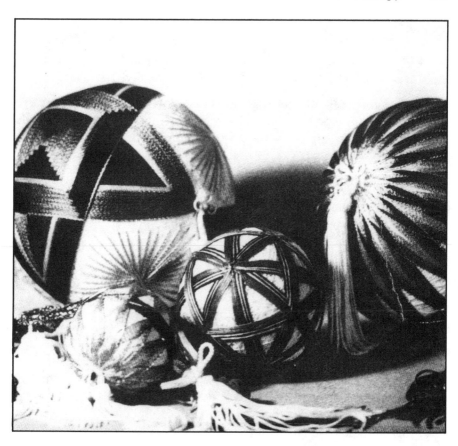

Yarn or Ribbon Balls

The beautiful items can be placed among plants to brighten a corner, hung from curtain rods to bring sparkle to any window, included in a centerpiece for a table, or even used as a toss item during physical activities.

In ancient Japan young mothers would start *temari* or "hand-rounds" for their daughters, winding one layer each year and often creating attractive patterns as the balls of colored material grew. When the daughters grew up, married, and left home, the mothers would give them the wrapped balls as symbols of their many years of loving care. The Japanese often used silk threads, but for older hands, yarn is easier to manipulate. Ribbon or silk embroidery floss can also be used.

Supplies

- An assortment of styrofoam balls 3 or 4 inches in diameter. (These can be purchased at craft shops or discount stores.)

- Varying shades of one-color yarn (light, darker, darkest) can present a beautiful gradation. Contrasting colors can also be used. Include a very light tone or white so that the colored pattern will show up.

- scissors (blunt end)

- A roll of masking or transparent tape to hold the yarn end when the work is put aside.

Instructions

1. Choose the color of yarn you like.

2. Begin by winding the yarn around a styrofoam ball, periodically changing the color or shade, and moving from lighter to darker colors and back again.

3. Wrap enough layers of yarn (or selected material) around the ball so that a distinct pattern will develop. The pattern will emerge depending on how the yarn is wrapped, so there is an element of surprise in the final pattern.

4. Tie a length of neutral-colored yarn to one "end" of the ball (where the colored lines cross over in the pattern, usually at the top and bottom of the ball). The ball is now ready to be displayed.

Needlepoint

The art of needlepoint has changed greatly from the time when it was associated mainly with chair cushions and kneelers. The development of plastic canvas, a loose-weave surface material that now comes in large sizes,* has opened up a whole new field of needlecrafts. If board and care residents are unfamiliar with needlepoint, they will be surprised at how easy it is to learn and how much fun it can be to make beautiful

---

*Needlepoint canvas is measured by the number of threads to an inch, thus a #12 canvas will have 12 threads to an inch.

items for themselves or others using the plastic canvas and a wide variety of colorful yarns.

The plastic canvas base, through which the thick thread or yarn is woven, comes in large sheets as well as pre-cut forms. A package of ten small pieces—round or square—is suitable for creating a variety of colorful and practical coasters to protect furniture from water marks and drink stains. Decorated coasters make an attractive and welcome gift for any host. The range of possibilities for needlepoint projects is limited only by the imagination of those who work with it: boxes to hold small personal treasures, holiday decorations, or beautiful frames for special photographs are just a few of the many items that can be created using plastic canvas and yarns.

The stitch techniques and instructions for making a large number of needlepoint designs can be found in any number of books on the subject. Your local library, craft store, or bookshop should be able to help you find just what you're looking for, both with respect to projects and the level of sophistication that can best complement the residents' needs and capabilities.

Intended Benefits

Working with yarn is an excellent source of exercise for the fingers, hands, and eyes. The mind is sharpened as different colors (and variations of the same color) are selected and a pattern is followed to arrive at a pre-determined design. Participants should work at a pace that is comfortable: arthritis sufferers or those whose movement is restricted because of painful muscles, bones, or joints should not overdo. As we are all aware, very detailed work can put a strain on the eyes if it is continued for too long. Those who participate in the needlepoint groups should be aware of their limits so they can rest when the need arises.

Individual creativity is stimulated as the cumulative skills developed through working with needle and yarn encourage residents to try more and more complex patterns. Decorative designs are created by varying the lengths of the stitches and by crossing over stitches, then repeating the technique. The pleasure that the elderly—both men and women—can experience from needlepoint is significant. By participating in this type of handicraft, residents gain a sense of personal satisfaction and fulfillment at their accomplishment, which helps to improve low self-image, bolster individual levels of confidence, and lift the spirits.

DRAWING

Drawing is an imaginative art that need not involve sophisticated technique or elaborate instruction; it's more important that the participants come to it with a genuine interest in expressing themselves. The tools can also be very simple: soft lead pencils (like those we all remember from kindergarten), a piece of pastel chalk, or a large crayon. Plain typing paper or photocopying paper can serve as the sketch surface. Some residents may prefer to have their own sketch pads so they can see how their skills develop and grow over time.

Like all skills, drawing takes practice to achieve proficiency. A felt stick designed for shading pencil lines can help accentuate a picture: dark shades push a subject back while light tones bring it forward. Gum erasers are handy for clearing away unnecessary lines or excessive shading.

Resident artists can begin by drawing an item from a picture: a simple flower (a daisy for example) as opposed to a more complicated form (a rose) and draw it from various perspectives—from the front facing the developing flower, from the side, from the bud stage, viewed partly closed or fully open. These viewing angles will help to prepare artists for drawing a bouquet of flowers later on, since bouquets show the same or several flowers in varying stages of development.

Whenever possible, use live models. Daisies can be obtained almost anywhere and at virtually any time of the year. If fresh flowers are not immediately available, silk ones best simulate the live plants.

A great variety of drawing tools are available both for those who are just starting out and the more seasoned artists. Colored pencils are useful for first-time artists, since they are not as messy as crayons or pastels. Pencils are also easier for frail hands to grasp. Using pencils, residents are better able to make fine lines, which may appeal to some beginners.

Felt-tip "brushes" are now available. The tip is rounded and can deliver as much or as little color as is wanted. Ordinary felt pens also come in a range of colors, and elders may enjoy using them.

Charcoal "pencils" in a variety of colors can also be purchased. They look like regular pencils but are really pastels encased in wood. Softer in consistency than the colored pencil lead, the charcoal variety crumbles more easily and will smear if brushed.

Encourage all residents to try their hand at drawing. Some will be very reluctant: like many of us, elders in board and care homes have been indoctrinated with the idea that "only artists can draw" or that they haven't any talent, both of which are destructive messages that are for the most part *just not true*. What is true is that different people will have different levels of talent. For some, drawing and painting hold little or no interest. They may prefer tinkering with machines, cooking, collecting, or some other activity. Some elders—especially those who must live in board and cares—find themselves limited as to the number and range of activities they can engage in, particularly when compared to what was possible before they moved into the facility. These residents must be encouraged to make the most of the limited space they occupy and the reduced capacities they now possess. As we said earlier, art can be a successful therapeutic alternative. Pain often slips into the background as artists become absorbed in what they are trying to accomplish.

PAINTING

The use of finger paints is often a splendid way to introduce beginners to the wonderful world of art. Standard water-based paints will not stain clothes or hands and can be washed off easily with the help of ordinary soaps and detergents. While safe to use and easy to clean up, finger paints are still messy, so if enough large men's shirts can be found in used clothing bins, the local Salvation Army Store, or donated by family members, cleaning up becomes that much easier. "Mother hubbard"-type aprons (those with full skirts plus a front bib that fits securely around the neck of the wearer) can also be used for this purpose. Who knows, maybe a generous beautician or supply house would donate used plastic aprons.

The colors and paper for finger painting can be picked up at any hobby shop, school supply store, and even in some well-stocked bookstores. Watercolors are odorless and easy to handle. A tiny bit of water can be brushed on crayon or pastel paints to blur or shade lines. Acrylic paint is popular and is remarkably close to oil-based paint in its effect. If oils are used, however, the painting sessions should be held outdoors or in a well-ventilated room; the turpentine and shellac needed when using this paint emit fumes that may irritate some people.

If board and care staff members are unsure about leading a drawing or painting group, then a volunteer teacher from an adult education department might be available to conduct it, or possibly someone from the art department of a local high school or college could help. If an art student can be found to assist, every effort should be made to arrange for the person to receive extra credit and/or a small stipend for this valuable service.

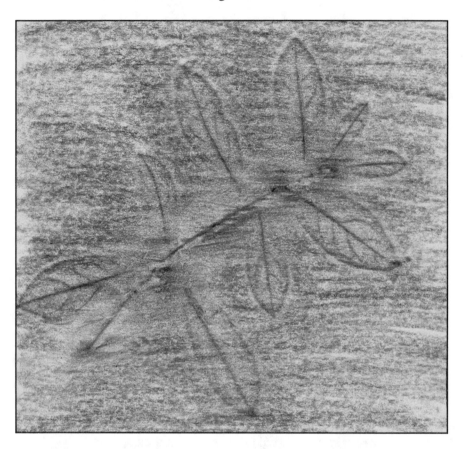

Videotapes on art instruction are available. Residents who are not visually impaired can watch a teacher on the screen and follow step-by-step instructions after the tape is over. One advantage of this format is that relevant portions of the tape can be replayed as needed to clarify a technique or to illustrate a point. Most television instructors prefer to have their audience watch first then attempt what they have been shown once the program has ended.

RUBBINGS

Impressions can be taken from an object by placing it underneath a thin sheet of paper and rubbing crayons or charcoal over the paper, pressing down to emphasize the covered object—hence the name "rubbings." Leaves with well-developed vein structures or "ribs" are a popular subject for this art form. The underside of the leaf may show up better. One or two large leaves or an arrangement of several smaller leaves, which have been affixed to an undersheet with transparent tape, works quite well. Very small leaves can be arranged artistically to give composition to the rubbing. Of course, ferns, small branches, embossed surfaces, and a host of other items can also serve as the raw material for creative rubbings in fascinating designs and patterns.

Supplies

- Gather leaves of various sizes and shapes: try to locate those with well-marked veins; seek out older, more mature leaves rather than new ones (many of which lack fully developed vein structures). The search for leaves can take place any time of the year but think what a beautiful outing it would make in the fall if the facility is located in an area where seasonal colors can be enjoyed.

- light-colored, standard-sized (8½″ × 11″ or 11″ × 14″) construction paper and newsprint

- crayons (the larger, thicker ones if possible)

- cellophane or masking tape to hold the leaves in place

Instructions

1. After gathering the leaves, spread them on a sheet of newsprint or on any surface that will allow you to hold them in place with bits of tape. When securing the leaves be sure to do so in the least intrusive manner, that is, tape only the stem and the tip of each leaf. You don't want to find an outline of tape on your rubbing! Alternatively, you can position the leaves, put the construction paper over them, and then paperclip the sides of the paper together. This should keep the leaves in place while preventing the need for tape.

2. Cover the leaves with a piece of light-colored or plain construction paper, then firmly rub over the top of the leaves with a crayon, a thick led pencil, or charcoal. Try varying the amount of pressure applied to alter the effect. Since the leaves can move a bit during this process, finish rubbing over one leaf before moving on to the next.

3. Lift off the finished rubbing. It is now ready to be mounted or framed.

Artists can learn a great deal about the structure of leaves, their functions, and life process while creating beautiful pictures.

CLAY OR CERAMIC SCULPTURE

As was mentioned when hand exercises were discussed earlier, working with play dough, salt and flour dough, potter's clay, or other ceramic clay is good physical therapy for the fingers, hands, arms, and shoulders. It also stimulates the sense of touch. Salt and flour dough is made from ingredients commonly found in most kitchens. The recipe is very simple:

> (Recipe can be duplicated as needed)
> 2 cups all-purpose flour (not the self-rising type)
> 1 cup iodized salt
> Enough water to make a firm dough
> Knead well until smooth and firm. Store in a plastic bag.

Residents can be involved in every step of dough preparation: mixing, kneading, and smoothing the dough until it is shiny and firm.

There are several books for beginning sculptors in the resource section of this chapter, any one of which will help board and care residents get started. The confidence level of the participants will improve as their knowledge of dough and clay work increases and they become more aware of the possibilities of this art form.

Making a Bowl

1. Take a small amount of dough and roll it out in a long, snake-like rope about ¼-inch thick. Keep rolling the dough until the diameter of the entire length of the rope is even throughout.

2. Coil this rope of dough into a tight circle. This will form the bottom of the bowl.

3. Roll out another rope of dough following the instructions in (1).

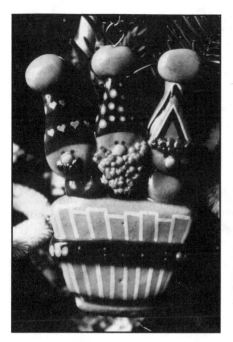 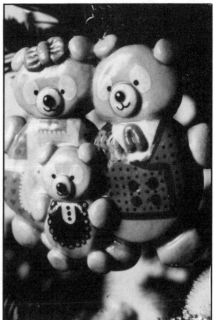

Courtesy of Family Circle, Christmas Helps; © 1981.

4. Take a second dough rope and place it on top of the outside rim of the dough coil that now forms the base of the bowl. Be sure that the dough ropes forming the side of the bowl fit tightly to each other and that there are no gaps or holes from which liquids could escape.

5. When the sides of the bowl are 2 or 3 inches high (or however high you decide to make them), smooth them with your fingers (with moistened fingers, one hand on the outer side of the bowl and one hand on the inner side, to close up these gaps), a stone, a piece of hard wood, or any hard surface until the sides are of an even thickness.

6. Let the bowl stand until thoroughly dry. If faster results are desired, it can be put in an electric oven at very low heat or in an unused gas stove (the pilot light will provide enough heat to dry the bowl).

Salt dough figures come out fairly light in color and are suitable for holiday ornaments and decorations, dolls, animals—the possibilities are endless. Small, useful items such as toothbrush holders, dry flower containers, pen/pencil holders, and even jewelry can be made from this dough. Flowers or designs can be painted on the dried bowl or animal shape. Salt dough sculptures can also be fired like other potter's clay: if a kiln is not readily available, ask a local school or ceramics shop if you might borrow theirs.

Intended Benefits

Any activity that requires the extensive use of hands, fingers, wrists, arms, and shoulders is very welcome, especially for residents who must remain inactive for long periods of time or who rarely move from their chairs during the day. Hand-eye coordination will also improve as participants become more adept at manipulating the dough and as their imaginations explore the possibilities for special creations.

HANIMALS

We have included the making of "Hanimals"—a word created by Mario Mariotti by combining "hand" and "animals"—under the heading of art activities because paints are used, even though it probably isn't, strictly speaking, "art." Nevertheless, the completed Hanimals are works of art. This is an activity that reinforces the sense of touch.

Making Hanimals can be viewed as both a variation and an improvement on the shadow pictures many of us recall from childhood—those primitive creatures that stalked the blank projection screen or an adjoining wall as light from a source behind us allowed the casting of shadows. Using water-based paints that wash off easily and the moving "eyes" found in craft stores (marbles or buttons can also be used), an amazing variety of animals can be made with just our hands. According to Hanimal creator Mariotti:

> The human hand is of great symbolic importance. With it we touch others, we bless, we make, we pray, we speak, we greet, we nurture. Early humans deliberately painted their hands on the walls of their caves. . . . Do not hesitate to roll up your sleeves and plunge into the paint. Let your imagination flower. . . . You can bring a whole world of new animals to life (as hanimals).[1]

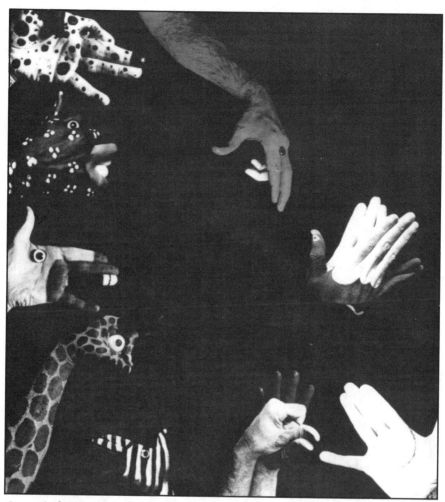

The waterbased paints can be applied to the hands with a brush, with cotton, or by dipping your hand into the color. Eyes can also be painted on or represented by toy "eyes" found in craft stores.

Method

1. Select the animal to be depicted. It can come from a picture or from your own imagination.

2. Practice posing your hands so that the animal is represented.

3. Color your hands. For example, to paint a zebra, first paint your hand white, then add black diagonal stripes.

4. Try using your Hanimals as props while telling colorful stories. The use of Hanimals lends itself to fanciful tales.

WOOD SCULPTURE

Some residents have many fond memories of whittling wood in their younger years. Board and care staff members may want to encourage these elders to return to this hobby, unless it represents a potential danger, or if residents' hands lack strength or shake too much. Even if they are not able to whittle or carve, they might enjoy making small wooden items like toys or bird houses. These activities require available work space where wood chips on the floor pose no immediate problems. In milder climates woodworking offers a delightful opportunity to enjoy the outdoors.

The feeling of working with wood is different from that of working with clay or dough. To lovingly sand and rub a fine piece of wood to give it that "sheen" is certainly a stimulating activity. It can also be a very creative one.

Woodworking may give male residents a greater sense of accomplishment, although many women fully enjoy handling fine woods. Since older men are often overlooked when art classes are proposed, working with wood might be a good way to get them involved. Keep in mind that residents should wear protective goggles and face masks when working with wood so that small chips and sanding dust don't pose a health risk.

Intended Benefits

The whole idea of engaging in arts and crafts projects as a form of therapy has only recently been recognized. Art therapists are only now being trained to begin working in the field of aging. Professional art therapists have found that intense concentration while creating a work of art, whether simple or complex, brings physical changes in the artist. One woman, for example, had tried every conventional treatment for arthritis yet could not find relief from its pain. After starting to work with crafts, over a period of two years she not only found relief from much of the pain but, because she was using her hands, she regained some flexibility in her fingers. Severe damage from years of arthritic pain and suffering could not be reversed, but the degenerative process and rigidity was eased considerably.

As a response to residents engaging in activities that give them a tremendous sense of accomplishment—they are creating something from within themselves—their brains secrete the pain-suppressing and pleasure-enhancing chemical endorphins that have been linked to "highs," not unlike the physical pleasure enjoyed by joggers or by those who meditate. Neuropeptides, another chemical secreted by the brain, stimulates the immune system. These are just some of the benefits that residents can obtain from creating an art object with their own hands.

NOTE

1. Mario Mariotti, *Hanimals: A Star and Elephant Book* (La Jolla, Calif.: The Green Tiger Press, 1982).

RESOURCES

Numerous craft books can be found in almost any bookstore as well as in every hobby shop and library. The level of activities chosen should be based upon residents' capabilities, and accompanied by easy-to-follow instructions. The Juvenile Books Department of your local public library is a good source for projects geared to beginners. These books also provide an idea of what kind of supplies will be needed.

Arts and Crafts (General)

Benton, Mary Ann, and Richard Bagwell, eds. *Teaching Creative Arts in Convalescent Hospitals.* Vista College, 2030 Milvia, Berkeley, CA 94704 (415) 841-8431.
Weisberg, Naida, and Rosilyn Wilder, eds. *Creative Arts with Older Adults: A Source Book.* New York: Human Sciences Press, 1984.

Thread Arts: Needlecrafts, Macrame, Etc.

Afghans, Leisure Arts, P.O. Box 5595, Little Rock, AR 72215.
Bonds, Cathy, Carol Millsap, and Jo Smity. *Macrame Purses: All Around Town.* Craft Publications, Division of Plaid Enterprises, Inc., 6553 Warren Dr. P.O. Box Drawer E, Norcross, GA 30091.
Christmas Projects for Plastic Canvas, Leisure Arts (see address above).
Leisure Arts, leaflet #153, (see address above)
Macrame: Start to Finish. Temple City, Calif.: Craft Course Publishers, Inc., Temple Craft Publishers, 1971.
Pesch, Imelda Manalo. *Macrame: Creative Knotting.* New York: Sterling Publishing Co., Inc., 1972.
Schwartz, Barbara. *Sewing with Yarn.* Philadelphia: J. B. Lippencott, Co., 1977.

Crafts Using Natural Products

Cutler, Katherine N. *From Petals to Pine Cones: A Nature Art and Craft Book.* New York: Lothrop, Lee & Shepard, Co., 1969.
Inouye, Carol. *Nature Crafts.* New York: Doubleday & Co., 1975. This volume includes instructions for crafts and sculpture using items easily found around the house or yard: stones, shells, driftwood, flowers, leaves, fruits and vegetables, cones and nuts.
Jordan, Nina R. *Holiday Handicraft.* New York: Harcourt, Brace, and World, Inc., 1966.

Ceramics and Clay

Gilbreath, Alice. *Slab, Coil & Pinch: A Beginner's Potter Book.* New York: William Morrow & Co., 1977.
Isenstein, Harold. *Creative Claywork.* New York: Sterling Publishing Co., 1969.
Payne, G. C. *Adventures with Clay.* New York and London: Frederick Warne & Co., 1967.

Miscellaneous Crafts

Cummings, Richard. *101 Masks*. New York: David McKay Co., 1968. With sound, basic knowledge and a lively, humorous style, the author presents diagrams and drawings to make this activity fun. Masks are not just for Halloween; they can be used for Greek or Japanese drama, or residents could have a masquerade party.

Holz, Loretta. *Mobiles You Can Make*. New York: Lothrop, Lee & Shepard Co., 1975.

Huff, Vivian. *Let's Make Paper Dolls*. New York: Harper & Row, 1978. This book describes many easy ways to create paper dolls. The photography is clear and helpful and the instructions are well thought out.

7

Music Therapy

In all its diverse forms—singing, listening to live or recorded concerts, playing an instrument, or discussing favorite performances by admired composers and musicians—music can be very therapeutic. It can be especially beneficial for those whose auditory sense is substantially intact. Music is a wonderful medium through which we can reach out to elders. Even those who are hearing impaired can "feel" the beat (rhythm), though it cannot be plainly heard.

Music is particularly effective for elders who experience depression, loneliness, feelings of isolation, memory lapses, speech impairments or slowing of speech, as well as physical and mental problems—in other words, the majority of those who live in board and care homes. Their hearing may be poor and their vision blurred, but many residents can still recall the songs they used to sing so many years ago. It is not surprising to hear visually impaired older adults sing several verses of favorite hymns from memory. Many elders remember songs that were popular when they were quite young, particularly if they enjoyed dancing to the melodies and singing the lyrics or had the good fortune to associate a romantic relationship with some special song. Sometimes a piece of music will evoke a sad or poignant memory and tears are shed; still, it is a healing act. Often a flood of memories surface as a song evokes sadness or joy; and if they bring tears, it may be helpful to share the reason behind them.

In this chapter, we present ways in which people who are not trained in music can use readily available resources. What we offer here are suggestions to get board and care facilities started in this direction. Maybe some of our ideas will trigger additional suggestions from residents or staff leaders.

Audio resources include recordings (records, cassettes, compact discs, and videotapes) to be used for sing-alongs. Hymns, music of the "gay nineties," and songs popular during and after the two world wars are especially familiar to most elderly residents. Mitch Miller, the popular conductor and choral leader, and others have recorded favorite folk songs and Christmas classics. Librarians should be able to help you locate the recordings, and most record shops carry a wide selection of music for the older audience. Well-known melodies could be purchased for the board and care library and thus made available year after year. Scan local television program listings for any concerts offered that focus on music of the twenties, thirties, forties, and fifties. When something of interest appears on the program schedule, residents could have an "Evening at the Concert," a special event set aside just for rekindling old memories of the music and the good times they knew so well. Local school bands/orchestras and community music or singing groups could be contacted about performing for board and care residents—or maybe for groups of residents from several facilities—at some agreed upon place (a local lodge hall perhaps).

Any musical activity can be therapeutic: it brings joy to the heart, exercises vocal cords and lungs, encourages deep breathing, and stimulates the mind's ability to record and retain information. Try to enjoy music every day.

INSTRUMENTS AND EQUIPMENT

Nearly every board and care facility will have one or more television sets. Some even have a video cassette recorder (VCR). But listening and viewing are passive activities; what is needed are ways to get the residents involved in what they are seeing and hearing. It is important to encourage those who listen to music to sing along, to join in the mood and get the feel of it—get them tapping their feet, clapping their hands, and swaying to the rhythm.

Many board and care homes lack the space or the financial resources to have a piano on the premises. However, we strongly urge all residential care facilities to consider purchasing a portable electronic keyboard. These instruments are programmed with built-in chords, tempos, and accompaniment, each of which can be recalled from the keyboard's computer memory at the press of a button. A keyboard is simple to learn, especially for those who may have taken piano or accordion lessons at some time during their lives. An accompanist can pick out the melodies and the keyboard will repeat them so that resident singers can follow the songs.

Percussion instruments, such as small drums, maracas, tambourines, bells, or chimes, can be purchased at any music store. Smaller versions of the above instruments can be found in toy stores or shops that specialize in audio equipment. *Better yet, residents can make their own percussion instruments. It can be an interesting craft project.*

Making Percussion Instruments

Fruit juice cartons or other cans/boxes that come with plastic lids will serve as the basic container for the instrument. Once cleaned and completely dry, the containers can be filled with dried beans, seeds, grains, or tiny pebbles. Varying the size, hardness, and amount of the "filler" will result in the shakers having different tones. With contact paper (the patterned, sticky-backed variety often used for lining cupboard spaces) residents can decorate the outside of these instruments. Not only is this plastic-coated paper attractive but it's also washable. Residents should use their imaginations; no doubt they will come up with some very inventive ways of personalizing their instruments and making them distinctive. There is one extra consideration to keep in mind: In this day and age of international concern over endangering our environment with overflowing landfills, these easy-to-make instruments help to recycle paper, plastic, and metal.

Cardboard cartons—such as the ones rolled oats come in—make splendid drums. So long as the hard plastic lid is not broken when the package is opened, these cartons provide the raw material for fine percussion instruments. After cleaning out the inside of the container, secure the lip with glue or sturdy tape, then wrap the side of the drum with contact paper or other decorative materials.

Stitch three to five small bells (like the ones found on pet collars) onto a heavy grosgrain ribbon or onto strips of colorful, sturdy fabric to give a real jingle to the percussion section.

The residents' choice of materials to make instruments is limited only by their imaginations, enthusiasm, and inventiveness. There are groups of "kitchen bands" who use ordinary household items to create a unique sound: e.g., wooden spoons on pot lids, old-fashioned washboards, hand-held crank egg beaters, and large jugs that make a deep resonating sound when air is blown across the top opening.

LET'S SING!

The people who publish *Reader's Digest* distribute a series of large-print song books whose themes are grouped according to historical periods (e.g., the gay nineties, the roaring twenties, etc.) or by type of song (e.g., holiday favorites, religious music, big band tunes, war songs, and ballads). See if your local public library subscribes to the series. Many music stores also carry these large-print song books.

If readable song books are not available, words could be printed by hand with felt-tip pens on ruled paper. If approached, a local high school music department might be willing to have its students create these song books as a class project. For singers, it is enough just to print the words in large letters so residents can follow along. In many instances, the elders are already familiar with the melodies or are instantly reminded as soon as someone hums a few bars.

The sheets of song lyrics should be in the same order as the accompanist plans to play; this way the residents can go through the songs one at a time without having to stop and search for the correct page. Older adults with vision problems or who are a little confused need a set routine. If the singing group meets frequently, vary the presentation slightly by starting from the back of the book and working forward, starting in the middle and progressing forward, or working your way from the middle to the back of the book.

The Accompanist

If the board and care has a piano or a keyboard, find a volunteer pianist to come in and play for the residents. If a piano or keyboard is not available, other instruments such as guitar, harmonica, or accordion can be used. Live accompaniment assists elders to follow the song and, more important, it brings someone into the facility from the "outside." This novelty always adds to the group's enjoyment. In addition, accompaniment for sing-alongs makes the homemade percussion instruments more fun to use. If a retired piano teacher or a volunteer from a nearby church cannot be found, maybe a music student would be willing to offer his or her services. Again, a small stipend will help ensure that the student keeps to the agreed-upon schedule (and it serves as a small token of the residents' appreciation for the person's time and effort). A practicing music teacher, choral director, or other volunteer professional may be willing to recommend a present or former student. A skilled musician can also accommodate the elders' vocal range by playing in a slightly higher or lower key.

If live accompaniment is not available, cassette tapes or records can provide the music for sing-alongs. Remember, for many communities, if fifteen residents or other participants join in the group, some school districts are able to provide an adult education teacher who would visit on a regular basis. (Of course, this suggestion may only be viable for larger residential care facilities.) An early-morning song or two can help start the day with enthusiasm, an after-breakfast boost to energize residents for up-coming activities. Music and singing are so very important to residents that they warrant a full block of time all their own. Morning songs are certainly valuable, but they are no substitute for a rousing sing-along hour later in the day.

Never discourage residents who cannot sing, who sing out of tune, or who have not sung in many years. They can join in by speaking the words in a normal tone of voice in time with the other singers. This saying or mouthing of the words should be done in a disciplined manner, maintaining the phrasing and rhythm of the song. In fact, it might prove interesting to try what is called a "voice choir": the group speaks the words of a poem or a short story, much like reciting Shakespearean plays or ancient Greek drama.

Getting into Position

Before actually beginning to sing, a short training session should be offered to give everyone an opportunity to speak the words aloud in proper sequence, to become accustomed to the timing—the beat of the music—and to get comfortable with proper breathing. Good singing begins with good posture. While seated in a straight-back chair, feet firmly on the floor, all participants should sit back with shoulders positioned a few inches from the back of their chairs; all heads should be up, making a straight line from the abdomen to the vocal cords. This erect posture permits a free flow of air, which is needed for singing. It is surprising how few people breath properly: most are accustomed to slouching in an easy-chair and breathing shallowly—the lungs are therefore never completely filled with fresh air.

Add Movement to Song

Residents can be encouraged to "swing and sway" while singing, listening to a melody, or mouthing the lyrics in time to the music. They can clap in time, tap their feet, or move and sway freely as they begin to "feel" the music. By moving to the music, elders exercise without even realizing that they are doing something beneficial for their bodies. No one has to tell young children how much fun it is to express themselves when music is played: they quite naturally begin to dance when they hear a catchy tune. But Western culture has placed social restrictions on this natural desire to dance, and "proper grown-ups" often insist that children sit still and remain quiet. In the generation(s) from which today's elderly emerged, the idea of moving to music was generally frowned upon. Some religious denominations even considered it sinful. One's upbringing is hard to overcome at times, but when residents are allowed to feel at ease and free to move about as they get caught up in the music, they might discover a new source of pleasure.

Residents who are wheelchair-bound or unsteady on their feet can still move to the music while seated, swaying from side to side, clapping their hands, or tapping their feet.

Intended Benefits

A vigorous period of singing forces the body to breathe deeply, bringing fresh oxygen into the system, thereby stimulating heart and lungs. Muscles in the chest, back, rib cage, and diaphragm are stretched, improving circulation in feet, legs, and arms. The psychological advantages of singing include personal satisfaction and enjoyment as well as group involvement. The mind benefits from the workout it gets recalling the words and the tunes.

CHOOSING THE RIGHT MUSIC

Some old familiar songs can be choreographed to incorporate a variety of body movements. Most of these songs, and the body motion associated with them, are nearly second nature to some residents:

"Jacob's Ladder" (using a climbing motion);

"Row, Row, Row Your Boat" (moving arms and shoulders in a rowing motion—divide the group and sing it as a round);

"Are You Sleeping?" (another round);

"He's Got the Whole World in His Arms" and "Kum Ba Yah (Come by Here)" invite sweeping motions of the arms;

"This Is the Way We . . ." (wash our hands, brush our teeth, etc.) suggests familiar, everyday motions.

Movement designed to accompany songs should be spontaneous and follow the words closely. No special training or background is needed to fit motion to the lyrics of some well-known piece of music. Movements should be free and a bit exaggerated or sweeping. This is an opportunity for residents to be expressive. Stretching should be encouraged as much as possible. American sign language, a system of hand gestures for communicating with the deaf, has motions that lend themselves well to movement with song:

"you" can be a sweeping gesture away from the body and toward another person, with index finger pointing;

"love" might be shown as a hugging motion with arms stretched across the chest;

"the cross" could be depicted by having one hand (say the left hand) held palm down with its little finger out away from the body while the right hand is held vertically (palm facing left) with the base of the little finger near the tip of the thumb;

"praise" could be shown as up-stretched arms, palms facing out.

In songs like "This Is the Way . . . ," the motion should complement the words. Teachers of elementary or kindergarten children are often well versed in these action songs. The board and care facility might want to invite a knowledgeable teacher to come lead residents in several of these songs. The lyrics for a variety of useful songs are provided in Appendix 7.

RESOURCES

Agay, Denes. *The Joy of Song.* New York: Yorktown Music Press, n.d. Easy piano arrangements with words and chords of popular, standard, folk, and holiday songs, among others.

Seeger, Ruth Crawford. *American Folk Songs for Children.* Garden City, N.Y.: Zephyr Books, Doubleday & Co., 1948. Contains many of the old favorites residents will remember from childhood.

John, Timothy, Peter Hankeyill, and Tom Ungerer, eds. *The Great Song Book.* Garden City, N.Y.: Benn Book Collection, Doubleday & Co., 1978.

8

Physical Exercise

We generally think of "exercise"—whether it be bicycling, tennis, jogging, swimming, or whatever—as vigorous, slightly unpleasant, or difficult. Clearly these activities are outside the capabilities of many board and care residents, but that doesn't mean elders in residential care facilities can't exercise at all. As we'll show in this chapter, even gentle, slow movements that an elder can make are beneficial for both body and morale. Exercise enhances mobility. To encourage more diverse movements, we have included several exercises to help board and care residents and staff get started. They include tension-reducing activities, exercises to loosen and tone muscles, and others designed to improve the cardiovascular system.

HELP IN LEADING ACTIVITIES

Contact your local parks and recreation department or similar agencies for the names of individuals who might be willing to come lead a weekly exercise group. A call to local high schools or colleges may well be rewarded with the names of students majoring in physical education or recreation who might be persuaded to conduct an exercise class on specific days. Work-study students who are capable of leading this kind of activity constitute another potential source of help. The board and care coordinator might suggest to the supervising high school teacher or college department that student helpers receive extra credit for their work. Perhaps a small fee could be paid to students as an incentive to meet at regular times and to be dependable.

Stress how important it is for these helpers to be prompt for scheduled meetings. Remind volunteers that residents and staff are expecting them; if they do not show up, the activity will have to be cancelled and many enthusiastic participants will be disappointed. However, it makes sense to cancel in case of illness. Volunteer leaders should not attempt to lead an exercise session if they are ill: even a simple cold can become a serious illness for frail elders, and in an enclosed facility the illness will spread rapidly throughout the resident population.

Another possible source of help are retired persons from the business community. Firms that keep in touch with their retirees are the best prospects. The utilities, local branches of large corporations, government agencies, and school districts often maintain contact with their retirees through newsletters. Organizations of retired doctors and nurses, lawyers, real estate agents, stock brokers, accountants, and other professional people usually meet with active members. Church groups, local chapters of the American Association of Retired Persons (AARP), senior center members, social and fraternal groups (such as the Lions, Rotary, Elks, Moose, etc.) have many members with varying skills. They are usually listed in the phone book. Contact the community relations department of various local corporations and ask to put a small article in their newsletter to recruit volunteers.

The recruitment of willing and loyal volunteers requires persistence and ingenuity—it's an ongoing process. However, such recruiting will pay off: well-chosen volunteers can help provide the health-enhancing activities that board and care residents need and that many states require of licensed operators.

Before attempting any of the exercises described below, residents should consult their physicians regarding appropriate levels of exertion and any recommended restrictions of movement that their doctors deem warranted. Physical activity leaders at residential care facilities can help in this process by providing a written exercise plan that the residents' physicians can approve or modify.

EXERCISES FOR THE MORE ABLE RESIDENT

Walking

For all those who are able, a walk in the fresh air each day, weather permitting, is energizing both mentally and physically. If an attendant cannot take the time to walk with ambulatory residents, possibly some arrangement can be made for high school or college students to volunteer their time after class. Retired persons could volunteer their time; even mothers with small children at home could bring their youngsters along for a walk with one or more residents.

When the weather does not permit a walk out of doors, older adults can walk around in a large room while swinging their arms gently. It's not the same as a good jaunt of several blocks, but this restrictive walking can be a stimulating alternative. Walking or marching in time to music can be a welcome change of pace, and it helps improve overall coordination. Go slowly, there's no need to rush. Even residents who require a cane or a walker can usually participate and benefit from this activity.

EXERCISE FOR SEMI- AND NONAMBULATORY RESIDENTS

Older adults who have difficulty walking can still exercise with the aid of a chair. These residents should sit in straight-backed chairs, preferably those with padded seats. Easy chairs or chairs with arms do not permit the required freedom of movement: elders will risk banging an elbow or an arm.

While considering activities that involve tossing or kicking, be aware that each resident has a different level of capability. Those who have had a stroke may find it difficult to throw or kick a ball as far as residents who have not suffered such a debilitating trauma. Residents with poor vision may not be as quick to discern direction or location. Activity leaders can compensate for this by casually moving closer before throwing to the less able, so that even the more restricted elders can be successful at the game or activity.

Everyone needs to feel like a winner occasionally. Reinforce, encourage, and praise participants—especially residents with severe disabilities. Give a cheer when someone overcomes serious problems or battles an obstacle to succeed in an activity. A kind word of praise makes that person feel good about accomplishing a goal. It also lets other participants know that, if at some future time they face similar obstacles, they, too, will be encouraged and praised, rather than made to feel embarrassed or inadequate. Every resident should receive one message loud and clear: "you are important and wanted."

Recommendations and Precautions

Those who lead exercise activities should keep the following in mind:

1. Avoid jerky or sudden moves, such as bouncing up and down while bending or stretching. Older muscles are easily pulled.

2. Begin a new exercise slowly; do it one or two times at first and then increase the number of repetitions as residents' abilities increase.

3. Rest a few minutes between exercises. This is a good time to do deep breathing to relax.

4. Encourage residents and praise their efforts: "Very good!" "You're doing great!"

5. Fill the time between exercises with light talk—jokes, riddles, short funny stories, or recent experiences. Encourage participants to share amusing anecdotes. Each new thought might trigger similar memories in others.

6. Laugh together. Many well-known publications have special features: *Reader's Digest* has a section called "Laughter Is the Best Medicine," and issues of *Modern Maturity* have a "Humor" page. It might be a good idea to collect bits of humor to keep on file. Chapter 9 offers a section on developing a "humor hour."

HAND MASSAGES

In recent years the art of massage has reached many people who enjoy having their hands, shoulders, or entire bodies skillfully touched. It releases tension and gives a sense of well-being. This loving gift of soothing touch is a great comfort to elders, too. They could even give each other a massage. Light Vitamin E oil, available at cosmetics counters, is generally used to soothe the skin. It is highly refined vegetable oil and lightly scented. It soaks into older hands immediately. This is very welcome as the skin of elders tends to be quite dry. One drop per hand is sufficient, but keep paper towels on hand to remove excess oil and to clear away any spills. Gently massage the back of the fingers, paying close attention to the base of the nails. Continue to massage the back of the hand, the wrist, and the arm at least as far as the elbow. Be very gentle; the skin of elderly persons is not only dry but fragile, since aging has reduced its elasticity. If a resident complains of pain, the masseur/masseuse may be rubbing too hard and should lighten the touch.

As their fingers, hands, wrists, and arms are being gently massaged, talk softly to the residents. This is a good time to hear any special concerns they may want to convey.

EXERCISES FOR ALL GROUPS

Toss or Kick Ball Games (While Seated)

Equipment

Though the materials available to the board and care staff may vary, the following is a good beginning for developing games that maximize participation and minimize strain.

Locate a couple beachballs or any air-filled plastic ball about ten to fifteen inches in diameter. If residents seem uncomfortable using these large items, try varying sizes of "nerf" or soft foam balls. Air-filled or nerf-type balls are safe for indoor play. You'll also need three seven- to eight-inch bean bags, a two-or three-gallon clean wastebasket or a container of similar size and depth for use as a "basket," and a large sheet of cardboard or thick butcher paper on which a bull's-eye target can be drawn. (Make the outer ring of the target about fifteen inches across and then a concentric circle inside, followed by a large black dot for the eye.)

Beginning the Exercise

Have the residents seat themselves in a circle around the edge of the room, leaving as much space across from each other as possible. If a resident prefers to stand, that's all right, but be alert to potential falls. The bones of older persons may be very brittle, and few things will undermine an elder's emotional or physical well-being more than confinement in bed as a result of a fractured hip or a broken leg.

Kicking a beach ball or other inflatable ball helps to exercise the legs, feet, and torso. Participants should bounce the ball lightly toward the center of the room. One resident will kick the ball across the circle to a fellow resident who, in turn, kicks it to still another. Begin slowly with a five-minute period and then gradually extend the exercise to ten or more minutes. Substitute the smaller ball and begin the exercise again.

Lifting legs so that feet make contact with the ball takes some coordination. Beyond the obvious workout for feet, ankles, legs, hips, and arms, and the improved circulation that should result, participants will enjoy a sense of competition. Muscles are exercised as the mind is stimulated to sharpen its reflexes. Usually this game is accompanied by considerable laughter, which is therapeutic in itself, for as Norman Cousins says, laughter "jogs the insides."[1]

To play *ball toss* the group must choose a leader who will be positioned in the center of the circle. The leader tosses one of the larger balls to each person in the circle in turn. One by one, the participants toss it back. During the first round the leader stands about three feet away from each player in the surrounding circle. For the second round those in the circle move back (or the leader moves closer to the center of the circle), widening the circle's perimeter until each player is about five or six feet from the center. The leader encourages the residents to aim their toss so that he or she can catch the ball. This is splendid exercise for hand, arm, shoulder, and eye muscles.

Toss games with balls or bean bags enhance hand-eye coordination. To encourage the use of hands, arms, body, and eyes in gauging distances by aiming for specific targets, leaders must change their distance from the players, either by moving closer or drawing farther away as the game proceeds.

If *catch* is the game of choice, residents should be in a circle with the leader standing about three or four feet away in the center. The leader tosses one bean bag at a time to a player. Each participant can then toss the bean bags, one at a time, back to the leader, who then moves on to repeat the exercise with the next person in the circle. When the leader has completed the entire circle of players, the group can then step back a few feet and repeat the tosses.

When playing *basketball* place the "basket" in the center of the room. Each resident is handed three bean bags and urged to aim and toss them into the basket. The leader will move the basket so it is about three or four feet away from all throwers on the first round. For the second and subsequent rounds, the players move back to increase the distance from which the bean bags are tossed/aimed toward the basket.

Remember the target we discussed above? Well, now it is time to try some "target practice." Position the target (bull's-eye) on the floor approximately six feet away from those participating in the game. Bean bags are then given to each player. When a participant's turn comes up he or she is encouraged to hit the bull's-eye. This activity, like basketball and the other toss games, helps hands and eyes work together while it stimulates sight, touch, and mental acuity. And don't forget—it's fun, too!

The following exercises are designed for specific body parts. Swinging the arms, rocking back and forth, bending in different directions, rotating the head and neck, and twisting at the waist are all valuable movements that help develop strength and flexibility. Swinging the arms is also part of T'ai Chi, which is included here as a separate activity because some consider it the best introduction to calisthenics. With few exceptions, these activities can be done while seated in a straight-backed chair or, if possible, while standing. Standing is preferable because it permits the easy and relaxed flexing of the knees. (We shall assume for the duration of this chapter that, unless otherwise indicated, residents are seated while exercising.)

Swinging the Arms

With your back remaining straight, arms dangling at your side, begin swinging them to and fro—relatively small swings that move the arms about six inches forward and then six inches back. After about twelve repetitions of this initial warm-up swing, widen your movement to waist height for about eight to ten repetitions, with a corresponding back swing.

Now lean forward and swing your arms from side to side in front of your body; then put both arms behind your back and again swing them from side to side. (This exercise is more comfortably performed while standing.) Allow eight repetitions of this last swing before gradually reducing the swinging motions to a complete stop.

You should begin to feel your shoulders relax; both shoulders and arms will probably tingle as blood circulates more vigorously throughout the upper body.

This is an easy and relaxing set of movements that can be done at a leisurely pace.

Rotation of the Head and Neck

Drop your head and neck forward so that your chin rests on your chest. Pause for a count of four. Then move your head slowly upward and to the right, as if to rest your chin on your right shoulder. Count to four. Now move your head back, tilting it as far as possible so your chin points straight up in the air. Pause again. Continue rotating your head to the left shoulder and then back to the forward position. Although residents should pause for a count of four at each of the four main positions, this exercise actually progresses in a continuous, slow rotation. Head and neck rotations should be done in cycles of four repetitions, beginning with movement to the right, then another four repetitions beginning with movement to the left.

Alternate Tightening and Relaxing

Lift your shoulders in an exaggerated shrug. With fists clenched, bend your arms at the elbow until both arms are tight against your body. Hold this position. Continue tightening your upper body, but this time clench your jaw, pressing upper and lower teeth firmly against one another; pursing your mouth; wrinkling your nose; furrowing your brows in a pronounced frown; and squinting your eyes shut. This position should be held for four slow counts, after which the muscles can be relaxed. Repeat this exercise two or three times. This quick tension release can make you feel better fast. It can be performed practically anywhere. What a great refresher after watching your favorite programs on television.

Mouth and Jaw

Drop your jaw as if it had come unhinged. The best way to accomplish this is to open your mouth very wide in a great, exaggerated yawn. After holding this position briefly (the usual count of four), close your mouth tightly and then relax. The huge yawn causes your throat and neck to open more than usual, thus relieving tension around the voice box. Follow this exercise with one in which you move your jaw from side to side, then in and out—each for a count of four.

Next, position your chin against your neck. Now attempt to wag your head slowly in a semicircular movement. The muscles in the back of the neck will pull slightly, loosening neck and shoulder muscles. This may be helpful in relieving tension headaches.

Fingers and Hands

Spread the fingers of both hands as far as possible. Hold this position for a count of four. Then clench your fingers together as hard and as tight as you can. Now relax your fingers by vigorously shaking your hands at the wrist. Shake them in all directions! Repeat this spread-and-clench action six or eight times.

While shaking your hands at the wrist, gradually lift your arms higher and higher until your hands are positioned over your head. After a slow count to four, lower your arms, but continue to shake your hands until your arms are down by your legs. Four full repetitions should be completed before taking a rest. This exercise will really loosen the muscles of wrists and arms.

Arms and Shoulders

Hold your arms in a clasped-wrist position (right hand holding left wrist while left hand holds right wrist), as if you are about to cradle a baby and rock it to sleep. For purposes of this exercise, you will be rocking your arms in an exaggerated motion minus the baby! Gently rock your arms and shoulders in a wide pattern from side to side, evenly and slowly, twisting at the waist, with your head always facing forward, bringing elbows as far back as your individual level of comfort permits. During this exercise you will experience a gentle pull on shoulder and back muscles.

"Rocking the baby" ten or twelve times in this manner gives enough "pull" on the back and neck to help loosen tight muscles. What a wonderful way to stretch arms, shoulders, and waist.

Feet, Toes, and Ankles

Seat yourself on a straight chair or, if possible, on the floor. If you are comfortable, try exercising barefooted or in stocking feet. This will provide a better range of moti n and more comfort. Do be careful, though; on floors that are not carpeted or at least rough surfaced to prevent slipping' the risk of falls is present. (On a comfortable day, an outdoor exercise period would be a delightful change of pace.)

With legs together and heels touching, spread your toes as far apart as possible, fanning them out, much the way you did with the fingers of your hand in the earlier exercises. Hold this position for a count of four and then relax. This exercise should be repeated four times.

With heels positioned on the floor, stretch the ball of each foot back toward your body at the instep. Hold this position for a count of four and then push your toes forward firmly for a count of four. Repeat each complete movement—backward and forward—four times, then rest. Feel the calf muscles in your lower leg tighten as the exercise progresses.

Now a bit of exercise for the ankles. Start by positioning your feet together, then lift them off the floor and slowly move both feet so that all your toes are pointing to the left as far as possible. Hold this position for a count of four and then return to the beginning position and rest a second or two. Repeat the exercise, pointing all your toes as far to the right as possible. Return to the starting position and rest. Do four repetitions of this side-stretching exercise.

As a slight variation on the above exercise, keep your feet together at the start, then bend both feet outward from the heel as the toes on your left foot stretch to the left and those on the right stretch to the right. Both variations will help to tighten the muscles above the ankles.

Another good exercise is to bring both feet together so that your big toes are touching. With toes pressed together, spread your heels apart as far as possible, hold the position for a count of four, and then bring them back together. Repeat this exercise about eight times.

Remember our hand exercises in which the hands were dangled at the end of the arm and then shaken vigorously? Well, now it is time to perform the same movement with your feet. Lift your legs up slightly and give each foot an invigorating shake: up and down and side to side, allowing each foot to move freely at the ankle. Now stop. Notice how relaxed your feet are? They are all warm and tingly.

Stretching Exercises

Knees, Calves, and Thighs

Start by lifting your left foot as high as you can, keeping your knee straight in front of you. Lift it slowly to a count of four, hold for four, and then lower it during a similar four count. Repeat this exercise three times. The same exercise should be done for the right leg.

Now, lean back in the chair with your feet on the floor. Slowly raise your left knee up to your chest (or as close as you can) during a count of four. Hold your leg in that position for another four-count (use your hands to hold your leg in place if this is more comfortable), then gradually lower your left knee to a count of four. Repeat this exercise three times. Now do the same exercise for your right knee and leg.

To exercise your hips, stand behind a straight-backed chair, your hands grasping the top of the chair-back. Rotate your hips by turning them to the left as far as you can and then to the right (much like the bump and grind routines of the old burlesque shows!). Now push your hips forward, pulling your stomach in; then push your hips back behind you as far as possible. Repeat this series of movements several times, then relax.

With your hands firmly grasping the chair back, hold out your left leg and shake it vigorously. Change to the right leg and shake it. Your upper body should remain still and facing the chair back.

These movements can help retain flexibility of hip joints and ease the stiffness that accompanies arthritis.

Deep Breathing and Bending

Exercises that focus on deep breathing and bending help to expand lung capacity as they stretch rib and back muscles. The exercises that follow should be entered into *slowly and deliberately.* They are designed to bring into play muscles that may not have been exercised in years. If every participant begins slowly and progresses at a comfortable pace, the number of stretching exercises can be gradually increased to suit expanded levels of endurance and physical flexibility. REMEMBER: DO NOT STRETCH IN A BOUNCING MOTION. Muscles that are not accustomed to being stretched in these ways can tear under the strain of abrupt movement. Besides, there is no need to hurry or rush—relax and enjoy the good feeling of your body in action.

Over and Under

To begin, all exercisers should be seated in straight-backed chairs, arms dangling loosely on either side. On a slow count of eight, and with arms remaining straight, slowly raise them directly in front of you until they are overhead as high as possible (a slight backward bending of the waist may be necessary to retain your balance). As your arms are being raised, your head and chin should also move upward (as though you are keeping an eye on your hands). Once your arms reach their highest point, hold this position for a count of four.

Now, gradually bring both arms back down during the same count of eight, but this time bend your waist until arms reach as far back as is possible, as though you are reaching for the back legs of the chair. At the midway point (the count of four) both of your arms should be positioned between your shoulder and your waist. By the time you end the eight-count, both arms should be below waist level and your upper body should be bent forward with your head resting at or below knee level. Hold this position for a count of four.

At the beginning of the count of eight to start either upward or downward arm movements, you should begin *inhaling* slowly and evenly. Upon reaching the point at which your arms are raised fully, you should hold your breath for a count of four. As the next count of eight begins to signal movement downward, you should begin *exhaling* slowly and evenly until your lungs feel empty by the time you reach the full downward position and have held your breath again for the count of four. This up-and-down exercise should be repeated four times.

Side Stretches

Beginning in the usual position, seated with arms dangling at your side, gradually lift your arms overhead, reaching up as far as possible. Slowly bend all the way to the right, keeping your arms straight overhead. Try not to bend forward or move so far to one side that you lose your balance. Hold this position for a count of four. Slowly return to the upright position and relax a bit; but keep your arms held high. Now bend to the left as far as you can and hold for a count of four. Return to the upright position.

Breathing is a significant feature of this exercise as well. While bending in either direction, residents should breath deeply and slowly. The rib muscles of older adults are not accustomed to being stretched in this manner so it might be wise to begin with only two bends in each direction, then gradually increase to four.

Upper Waist and Torso

During a slow count of four, lean over until your chest rests on your knees, or as close as you can come to this position. Your shoulders should be dropped in a relaxed way and arms should hang loose. Hold this position for a count of four. Now, during another full count of four, gradually return to an upright position. This exercise should be repeated four times.

Waist Twist

All participants should be either seated or standing, whichever is most comfortable. First, with your right hand clasp your left arm above the elbow; then with your left hand clasp your right arm above the elbow. This position might remind you of the dignified stance of an Indian chief, or a variation on the position used in the "rock-a-by-baby" exercise described earlier.

With arms and hands in this position, slowly turn to the right as far as you can and then pause. You might be able to go a bit farther by turning your head in the same direction as your twist and looking back at something behind you. Hold this position for a count of four, relax, and then return to the beginning position. Repeat the exercise, but this time go to the left as far as you can, looking for the same object/person you located behind you last time.

Throughout this exercise you should feel a refreshing but gentle pull on your waist and back muscles.

T'ai Chi

In our introduction to this chapter, we mentioned that T'ai Chi is one of the oldest forms of exercise. The form currently being taught to older persons is a gentle adaptation of the Asian martial art, though it includes none of the more abrupt movements. Basic movements are slowed down considerably to resemble a smooth, flowing dance (even though, for the most part, residents can be in a seated position while performing the movements). T'ai Chi periods are physically stimulating yet emotionally relaxing times of meditation.

Each of the movements that follow will help to stimulate a specific set of muscles. Residents will find that after engaging in T'ai Chi their fingers and feet tingle with the sensation of fresh blood coursing through their veins. The positions for hands should be followed with the eyes (try not to move your head unless it is part of a given exercise). The point of T'ai Chi is to strengthen muscles as well as the participants' control over them.

One added dimension to T'ai Chi is its use of the memory and imagination to assist in the description of movements. The point of naming the various exercises is to help residents keep an image in their minds, and this, in turn, brings certain muscles into play.

Catching and Dropping a Ball

Begin with your feet flat on the floor. Put your left foot forward. Imagine you are gathering air into a ball over your left shoulder. Slowly move it outward in a circle, leaning slightly over your left foot as you bring the "ball" in front of you at chest level. Turn your palms down and let the ball fall quite naturally, then begin to gather another air ball. Carry it toward your right shoulder in the same circular motion until it, too, is at chest level. Turn your palms down and allow this "ball" to fall as well. From left shoulder to right and back again is all one continuous movement for eight complete rounds. Try to keep your eyes on your hands as much as possible: this focuses attention on the movement and also prevents outside distractions from interfering with your concentration. All of this action should be carried out in a smooth, continual, uninterrupted motion. Move as slowly as you can. This increases your ability to control your motions.

Big Bass Drum

With hands out in front of you, palms facing and spaced approximately twelve inches apart, lift them together as if to trace the rim of a large bass drum that one might see at a parade. This drum will be positioned on your lap. Trace the outer rim of the drum by moving your hands toward you at about eye level, then move them downward against you, over your lap, and outward again. Repeat the circle eight times. Let your body sway forward and back as you circle the drum. Now bring your left foot forward: this will allow you to make the perimeter as large as possible, which will help you use your arm muscles more effectively. After eight forward repetitions, stop the circular movement, breathe deeply, and repeat the movements in reverse, this time with your right foot extended. Repeat this cycle of forward and backward movement three or four times and then rest.

Push and Pull

"Push out the old air, pull in the new." With one palm held out as if to signal "Stop," extend your hand and arm as far as you can. The palm of your other hand should be turned toward you, pulling air inward as though you were trying to bring energy from the air into your body. Simultaneously, one hand and arm should be pushing out while the other hand and arm is pulling in during a continuous movement of about eight repetitions (eight times out, eight times back). Rest and breathe deeply.

Mountain High

Begin with arms and hands widely extended at hip level, palms facing down. Slowly draw your hands inward, palms facing, while your arms rise up to form the sides of a large mountainlike cone. At the summit your hands should be about twelve inches apart. Hold that position for a count of four and then reverse the movement until your hands and arms are back to their original position. Complete about eight mountains.

Valley Low

This exercise is the reverse of mountain high. Begin again with hands and arms widely extended at hip level, palms facing down. Slowly, bring your hands up and toward the center so that the thumbs of both hands are just about at eye level. Gradually move your hands and arms down and away from your body below hip level, and up again to carve out two big valleys. Keep your motions steady and even, and complete eight repetitions.

Football Ellipse from Side to Side

Imagine you are holding a football over your left shoulder. Your fingers should be spread apart and bent as though you are grasping both sides of the ball. Sweep the ball down in a circular motion in front of your waist, then move up to your right shoulder, crossing over in front of your face, and back again to your left shoulder. In this manner you will be making an elliptical path with the ball. If you choose to stand while performing this exercise, then raise your knee high and take one step to the left during each of three repetitions. If you are sitting during the exercise, then sway as you make the ellipse. After three repetitions, pause and take a deep breath.

Now, do the same exercise in the opposite direction. This time begin with the ball over your right shoulder, swing it down and toward the left, in front of your face, and back again to the right shoulder—three times. This completes one set of the football swings. One set of these movements constitutes three times on the right and three times on the left. Participants are encouraged to do four sets.

Passing Clouds

This is a slow, dancelike exercise in which the upper torso is turned as far to the left and to the right as possible while the hands move in cloudlike patterns across the upper and lower body. It is designed to stretch the muscles over the rib cage and those of the waist.

Position your hands at waist level with both palms facing in, the little finger of your right hand resting atop the thumb of your left hand. Turn your shoulders and arms as far to the left as you can, twisting at the waist while keeping your lower body facing forward. During this turning movement, bring your right arm and hand up in a counterclockwise motion so that you are looking directly at the crease lines of your palm at just the time you are turned fully to the left. At the same time, your left hand should be moving in a counterclockwise pattern in front of your lower body in order to be in position to come up and be the "cloud" at the point at which you reach the farthest twist point on your right. As you start to turn to the left again, your left hand and arm begin to descend and your right hand and arm start ascending until your right hand is positioned in front of your face as you reach the farthest point of the twist leftward. Keep your eyes on the hand that is passing before your face. This makes the pull on the back and rib muscles that much more beneficial.

Try not to have any break in your movements. Continue to pass the right then the left hand in front of your face about eight to twelve times, each time making an oval pattern with your hand. When you have finished this exercise, stop, breathe deeply, and relax. This exercise is ideal for those who have a bit of trouble sleeping at night.

We encourage all residents of board and care homes to participate as much as they can in well-planned physical exercise groups. You'll feel better, sleep better, have a brighter outlook on life, and enjoy the company of friends. Your pleasure and enjoyment can be significantly enhanced if music is added to the exercise experience. There is much to be gained by a good workout—at any age!

RESOURCES

Games

The following children's game books are listed here because these games are often simple and easily adapted for elders with disabilities.

Cole, Ann, Carolyn Haas, Elizabeth Heller, and Betty Weinberger. *Children Are Children Are Children.* Boston: Little Brown, and Co., 1978.
McWhirter, Mary E. *Games Enjoyed by Children Around the World.* American Friends Service, XEROX Education Publications, 1970.

Physical Exercise

Berger, Bonnie G. and Bradley D. Hatfield. *Exercise & Stress*. New York: AMS, 1987.
Flatten, Key, et al. *Exercise Activities for the Elderly*. New York: Springer, 1988.
Jamieson, Robert H. *Exercises for the Elderly*. Hillside, N.J.: Enslow Publishers, 1982.
Lederach, Naomi, et al. *Exercise as You Grow Older*. Intercourse, Penn.: Good Books, 1986.
Meyer, Francis D. *Exercise Designed for the Aging*. Munster, Ind.: FDM Distributors, 1985.

Miscellaneous

KOOSH BALL

This is an inexpensive, squishy ball constructed of what looks like cut up rubber bands that have been made into a loosely formed ball. It can be tossed, squeezed, or just shoved around. When touched it moves in a very lifelike way. It can help those with arthritis increase the flexibility of fingers, hands, and arms, increase dexterity and endurance, and enhance one's sense of touch. KOOSH BALLS can be found at many toy stores and are manufactured by OddzOn Products, Inc., P.O. Box 1590 Campbell, CA 95009.

9

Miscellaneous Activities

In this chapter, we describe many activities that help to exercise the mind, the memory, and the emotions. The activities are enjoyable not only for board and care residents, but for volunteers and the staff as well. They are designed to be beneficial without necessarily having a formal place within any specific category of "therapy."

The best way to enjoy most activities is to enter into them with gusto and enthusiasm. Don't get bogged down trying to figure out exactly what type of therapy is being engaged in at this or that moment. We have listed the intended benefits of various activities at the end of each description so that staff or volunteer leaders will have some broad goals to work toward.

In considering the activities below, or any of the others described in this volume, readers should not limit themselves to what we have suggested. It is our hope that activity coordinators will develop their own ideas for stimulating and enjoyable programs, which are both within their ability to offer and within the capabilities of the residents they serve.

SLIDE PRESENTATIONS

Many people like to travel and a significant number of them take high-quality photographs of the countries, cultures, and peoples they have visited. Those who consider photography their hobby usually are quite pleased to come to a board and care at some conveniently scheduled time to present their slides of foreign or domestic travels. If the community has a camera club, then a board and care staff member might be able to contact a willing photographer whose work would be of interest to residents. Inquiries placed with local camera shops or neighborhood stores where film is sold and developed could prove helpful; or try contacting those who teach photography courses at universities, community colleges, or even adult education classes at high schools—they may know of hobbiests who display their work. It often pays to check with the men's and women's clubs of local churches. Often these organizations will be able to suggest one or more of their members who has shown various slides to community groups. A local librarian may also be able to assist, since often the main library or any one of its branch locations might call upon those in the community who travel to provide similar presentations.

We suggest that all photographs or slides be pre-screened before they are shown to residents. It's wise to be sure that the presentation is on a subject likely to interest, and possibly even challenge, those who choose to attend. This screening will also give the staff an idea of how long the presentation will last. Some subject areas are best suited to a shorter program, while for others it would seem that the residents could watch for hours.

Intended Benefits

It is often said that travel broadens the the mind. But for those who are no longer physically able to travel, vicarious adventures are still possible through slide presentations. Regularly scheduled slide shows featuring different countries, resort locations, or special hobbies keep residents interested and involved in the "outside" world. Their questions about the pictures, the locations, or the history and customs of a region can stimulate their imaginations and bring back a flood of memories about their own travel experiences of years ago. The enthusiasm and energy generated by these programs will challenge their minds with interesting information about foreign cultures and customs and excite curiosity.

A HUMOR HOUR

As we have seen time and again in this volume, the mental attitude of residents is an important factor in maintaining their physical well-being. Laughter that naturally emerges from pleasurable activities stimulates the body's production of chemical endorphins, nature's own pain-killers. Norman Cousins called laughter "jogging for the insides." A hearty laugh can be vital for our general well-being.

A "humor hour" or "laughter session" can be scheduled into a board and care's weekly activities. These sessions should be planned to meet the emotional needs of as many residents as possible. Of course, laughter is a universal response and should be encouraged during all appropriate activities. Its therapeutic value need not wait for the scheduled time of a humor hour.

It Takes Some Planning

There is no limit to the kinds or types of devices one can use for humor sessions. For example, videotapes of legendary comics are perfect: the Marx brothers, Lucille Ball ("I Love Lucy"), Jackie Gleason and Art Carney ("The Honeymooners"), Bob Hope's old road movies, the "Jack Benny Show," Charlie Chaplin, Buster Keaton, the Keystone Cops, Laurel and Hardy, the Three Stooges, Spanky and "Our Gang," Abbott and Costello, the old "Show of Shows" with Sid Caesar and Imogene Coca, Red Skelton, and so many others. In most cases, residents will recall having seen the work of some or all of these comic figures. Along with the laughter, there will be many fond memories of afternoons spent at the local theater with the great stars of silent films and later the "talkies." In fact, try recreating this nostalgic atmosphere by serving popcorn, soft drinks, and candy bars.

Animated cartoons are also available and will lighten the heart. The early efforts are particularly fascinating: though they are in black and white, the humor and slapstick is timeless.

Books of humor written by such authors as Mark Twain, Will Rogers, Robert Benchley, Erma Bombeck, and others can be read on a continuing basis and spread over several sessions. One of the more recent authors that residents might enjoy is Robert Fulghum, whose book *All I Really Need to Know I Learned in Kindergarten: Uncommon Thoughts on Common Things*[1] is a charming collection of essays that will evoke tears and laughter, often at the same time.

Investigate the humor section of the local public library to find old and new favorites. Most libraries have record collections that circulate, which may include recordings of live performances of stand-up comics: e.g., Myron Cohen, Jackie Mason, "Lonesome" George Goble, Shelley Berman, or releases of the old radio programs of George Burns and Gracie Allen, Amos and Andy, and others.

Reader's Digest has various sections offering funny stories, unusual experiences, or amusing one-liners. Keep an eye out for these. Often major magazines and newspapers have very funny cartoons. Clip these out and share them with residents.[2]

Making Use of Volunteers

It is always a good idea to recruit and train volunteers to come in and lead these laughter sessions. High school and college drama departments, youth groups, and people who work in senior citizen centers can be valuable sources of volunteer leaders.

Do keep in mind that just as humor often changes from culture to culture, much of what is thought to be humorous changes from generation to generation. Prospective volunteers should have comedic interests similar to those of the majority of board and care residents; otherwise, the volunteers will not be able to appreciate or properly convey the humor of the material being presented.

Develop a flyer that describes your intended activity. Identify the facility and list your name and number so that prospective volunteers have a specific person to contact. Incorporate a comical cartoon or picture in the flyer so that it attracts attention. A high school or college art department might be willing to help develop and design the flyer as a class project.

Meanwhile, back at the board and care, post written announcements for the humor session well in advance of the first meeting. Describe your program several times before the first session. Introduce your volunteer leader(s) to all residents. Mealtime is often a perfect occasion to make such announcements. Why not invite the volunteer to share the meal with residents? If a staff member is leading the session, let residents know well beforehand.

Preparing for a Humor Session

1. Review the following "Dos and Don'ts" with volunteers or staff members (these are taken from *Humor: The Tonic You Can Afford,* pages 17–18):

Some Dos

- *Be enthusiastic.* Know what you are aiming to do with your humor time. Don't be half-hearted. Know that the residents will receive positive benefits from your efforts.

- *Be patient and understanding* of residents' lack of experience in opening up to you and revealing their emotions. Take time to let them speak out. Don't rush on if someone is trying to get a point across. Be supportive of their efforts.

- *Be clear* about your purpose. You want to interact with residents, not entertain them.

- *Observe* residents' reactions. Note their remarks and/or the sharing of personal and very meaningful experiences.

- *Be prepared* to add a humorous touch to a situation where it is appropriate, but be sensitive that you do not intrude.

- *Smile, smile, smile!!*

Some Don'ts

- *Don't forget that the purpose of the session* is to get residents to laugh. Don't force the issue: to be beneficial, laughter must be spontaneous, not artificial.

- *Don't push* residents beyond their level of comfort.

- *Don't be inflexible.* Relax and enjoy this time together. Fortunately, there is no right way or wrong way to proceed. Each group will have its own pace and its own limits.

- *Don't be disappointed* if everyone doesn't want to participate right away. If those who do come to the session enjoy the time they spend, they will gladly relate their experiences to others and your group will grow.

- *Don't show favoritism.* Some people are more outgoing than others. Although there is probably a little bit of "ham" in all of us, some people will appear shy, withdrawn, and a bit reluctant to participate freely. Give them time. The more sessions they attend the more likely it will be that they will begin to express themselves. The acceptance of the group builds confidence and a willingness to take risks.

2. Try conducting a brief role-playing session with group leaders/volunteers before the first humor hour. Have some volunteers play the part of resident participants and others play the part of group leaders. Try to make this "dry run" as realistic as possible so that potential problems can be anticipated and dealt with.

3. Select the ideal location as well as alternative locations for the sessions. If the facility is small and all activities take place in some communal area, be sure that it is a comfortable, sunny, cheerful place. Put up posters, blown-up copies of cartoons, or other decorations that will bring a smile to residents' faces.

4. Gather pictures that have the potential to bring out laughter. Check the daily newspapers and any magazines. Don't overlook advertisements: agencies are experts at presenting ordinary ideas in a humorous manner. Librarians might have bright posters that can be checked out for use during a humor session. Books and posters depicting pet-owner look-alikes are especially appealing.[3]

5. Have refreshments: cookies and coffee/tea to create a relaxed and friendly atmosphere. Encourage residents to share a joke, a funny story, or a riddle. Riddles are particularly good because they force us to think, to associate ideas.

Intended Benefits

Norman Cousins found that two hours of hearty laughter gave him twenty minutes of freedom from a very painful illness. Board and care residents may also gain some relief from their aches and pains during times when their attention is diverted from ailments and directed toward interesting activities—and laughter can be quite a diversion. In addition, and often of far more importance, is the sense of being wanted by a group: this in itself has significant therapeutic value. In these important ways, elders find their mental and emotional health enhanced by humor sessions.

GARDENING AS THERAPY

Gardening is a sensuous and rewarding activity. Few hobbies offer such visible rewards as planting and nurturing flowers and vegetables. Handling soils of varying textures, choosing among seeds of different shapes and sizes, and immersing oneself in a rich variety of plants and seedlings can stimulate the sense of touch. The smell of earthy, wet planting mixtures, the scent of certain plants, and the aroma of developing fruits and flowers combine in a cornucopia of delights that bring to the surface wonderful memories of tending flowers or vegetable gardens years ago. Seeds or starter plants are lovingly nurtured, new growth is observed and tended to, and mature fruits or flowers are harvested.

Don't pass up a wonderful opportunity for residents to express their personalities and creativity just because of some notion that older adults in residential care facilities cannot garden—of course they can! Many city-dwellers enjoy gardening with planters and pots. With care and planning, residents can prepare soil, plant seeds and seedlings, and harvest a bountiful crop of vegetables, flowers, or herbs. This health-enhancing activity can be enjoyed on a patio, but it can also be adapted to accommodate the needs of those who must remain indoors.

Gardening has both immediate and long-range benefits:

- the exercise and mental stimulation

- the fun of preparing and eating the fruits of one's labors

- enhanced self-esteem.

The responsibility of caring and tending, weeding and fertilizing provides the opportunity for residents to feel useful and needed.

Gardening Materials

Suitable containers for planting will vary according to their size and type, availability (Will they be purchased, donated, or recycled from some existing container not initially intended for plants?), the specific needs of the gardeners, and the growth requirements of the plants. It is important that there be ample depth for root growth (one to two feet of soil should be adequate). Residents can use large metal drums that have been halved lengthwise, or any large container capable of holding between fifteen and twenty gallons of soil. Gardening can also be done in small or large flower pots available in terra cotta, plastic, or metal.

Prepare the container for adequate drainage. Nothing is more disheartening than to have plants die because the roots rotted as a result of poor drainage. This is easily corrected if pebbles or very small pieces of broken clay pots are placed at the bottom of the containers before they are filled with soil. Even wire mesh or fiberglass screening positioned over the holes in pots will work well enough. If the large drums are being used, bore holes in the bottom to allow for drainage, then fill with soil mixture and ready them for the plants. Inexpensive plastic dishes can be used to keep spilled or drained water from damaging furniture or floors. If the facility offers ceramics classes, residents could create these receptacles for overflow and other gardening items, such as the "self-feeders" that allow water to seep into the soil gradually.

A wide assortment of gardening tools is available, but for many jobs old spoons and spatulas work just as well. Old table knives can be used for making small holes to plant seeds or cuttings, and old wooden spoons or popcicle sticks can serve as handy poles and tools, as do large forks, prongs, or forceps.

Those who enjoy both needlepoint crafts and gardening might like to make macrame plant hangers out of heavy yarns, cord, or rope. These hangers will allow residents to have house plants in their rooms, which will help keep the air clean and fresh.

Nurseries and the garden centers of many stores carry packs of seedlings that are ready to transplant. These starter plants will help to capture residents' initial interest in gardening. Later they can plant the seeds of fast-growing vegetables and flowers, observe the sprouts as they break the surface of the soil, and tend the maturing growth. Consider conducting a group outing to a nursery: there are many fascinating choices for those who get hooked on gardening.

Some plants grow quite well from runners of existing plants. The spider plant is a perfect example. Other plants also do well if a cutting or a segment of an existing plant is potted and given time to root—Viennese Bridal plants and philodendrons are good choices—but many others can be potted and grown in much the same way and with very little effort.

Once residents have caught the gardening bug, many may wish to attend gardening shows, flower shows, botanical gardens, horticultural exhibits, or garden centers that have special displays of seasonal plants.

Potpourri

Creating fragrant potpourris is a delightful way to combine outdoor and indoor activity. Residents can gather sweet-smelling leaves and flowers and bring them indoors to dry in a cool, dimly lighted place. The dried items can be mixed with other fragrances, such as clove, dried citrus, cinnamon, or concentrated scents to form wonderfully aromatic combinations. Rose petals are perfect for potpourris because they retain their delicate fragrance even after being dried. Here's a hint: try the older varieties of roses—such as the American Beauty Rose—since they are more fragrant than the newer varieties. Combinations of conifers, needles, and bark can be combined to create a seasonal scent. And, of course, you can buy cedar bark.

Once the dried components of a potpourri are mixed, store them in a tightly covered jar. The fragrance of this jar of flowers, herbs, and leaves can be enhanced by adding a small amount of aromatic oil, which can be found in craft and candle shops. Once the oil has been added to the potpourri, store the jar in a dark place for about six weeks before using it; occasionally, shake the jar to blend the mixture. Small squares of thin, but tightly woven silk, chiffon, cotton, or linen can be filled with the potpourri. Then the corners and sides can be brought together and tied with a colorful ribbon.

ADOPT-A-GRANDPARENT

Throughout the country there is national program called "Adopt-a-Grandparent," which seeks to develop and nurture a personal relationship between one elderly person and some "outside" person or family. Such a program is particularly beneficial to older persons who have outlived their own families and friends or who have never had a strong circle of supportive friends or relatives. With the help of Adopt-a-Grandparent many discouraged, debilitated, and depressed elders are getting a new lease on life.

"Adopters" range from caring individuals to families, youth groups (e.g., Camp Fire Girls, Girl Scouts, Boy Scouts, 4-H groups, school service clubs), college groups (e.g., sororities or fraternaties), church groups, or social and fraternal organizations (e.g., Elks, Moose, Lions, Masons, etc.). Those who adopt a board and care elder visit regularly to talk, read together, or write letters for their "grandparent." Those who visit the visually impaired might read a chapter or two of a particular book each week. Before each new chapter is read, the visitor and the grandparent could recollect the substance and story line of the book up to the point at which that week's reading is to begin.

Other "adopters" share interesting articles in newspapers or magazines, while some keep in touch through telephone reassurance—calling several times a week to let their "grandparent" know that a caring person is interested in how the elder is getting along. Still others who adopt grandparents might take a resident on an outing: maybe to dinner, for a walk in the park, or to a movie. Some do small chores for their "grandparent": go on errands, drive the older person to the doctor, or accompany their elder to appointments. Though nothing will completely replace lost family members or departed long-time friends, adopting a grandparent can show our elders that someone cares and wants the older person to be a part of their life.

We wish we could put into words the joy and pride that board and care residents feel when someone from outside the facility takes the time to demonstrate interest and concern for their welfare. Feelings of personal self-worth and importance begin to increase when an older adult knows that someone really does care. Mild and even deep depressions can be replaced by a revitalized look and a true zest for living. For those who are alone in the world, programs like "Adopt-a-Grandparent" can be a vital point of contact with the outside world.

NOTES

1. Robert Fulghum, *All I Really Need to Know I Learned in Kindergarten: Uncommon Thoughts on Common Things* (New York: Villard Books/Random House, 1988).
2. Andrus Gerontology Center, *Humor: The Tonic You Can Afford: A Handbook on Ways of Using Humor in Long-Term Care* (Los Angeles: University of Southern California, 1983).
3. Editors of *Spy* magazine, *Separated at Birth?* (Dolphin Books/Doubleday, 1988)

RESOURCES

Humor

Andrus Gerontology Center. *Humor: The Tonic You Can Afford: A Handbook on Ways of Using Humor in Long-Term Care.* Los Angeles: University of Southern California, 1983. Offers step-by-step instructions on beginning to use humor as a way to stimulate sensory functioning among elders.

Breathed, Berke. Creator of the cartoon "Bloom County," which is now included in such paperback collections as: *Bloom County: Loose Tails* (1983), *'Toons for Our Times* (1984), *Penguin Dreams and Stranger Things* (1985), and *Bloom County Babylon: Five Years of Basic Naughtiness* (1986), all of which are published by Little, Brown and Company. (These funny and irreverent cartoons feature Breathed's main character, a penguin, who exemplifies all of us in our dreams and in our problems.)

Editors of *Spy* magazine. *Separated at Birth?* New York: Dolphin/Doubleday, 1988. (A small paperback featuring look-alike pictures of pets and their owners and famous people look-alikes.)

Fulghum, Robert. *All I Really Need to Know I Learned in Kindergarten: Uncommon Thoughts on Common Things.* New York: Villard Books/Random House, 1986–1988.

———. *It Was on Fire When I Lay Down on It.* New York: Villard/Random House, 1988.

(These collections of short essays cover many topics and are written in a humorous style. Fulghum's books can be used as mental therapy and in times of spiritual meditation or worship.)

Trese, Patrick. *Penguins Have Square Eyes.* New York: Holt, Rinehart, and Winston, 1962. (Trese is a script writer who was sent to Antarctica with cinematographer Bill Hartigan to record the building of facilities for the International Geographical Scientists group who were going to study conditions in the South Pole region. It is a fascinating adventure story told with much humor. It's a sample of the kind of book that can be read to a resident over several visits.)

Gardening

Baker, Sam Sinclair. *The Indoor and Outdoor Grow It Book.* New York: Random House, 1966.

Paul, Aileen. *Kid's Gardening.* Garden City, N.Y.: Doubleday, 1972.

Readers Digest Association. *The Magic and Medicine of Plants.* New York: Readers Digest Press 1989. (This volume gives many of the medical uses for plants. It is a fun book that contains the history, growth requirements, as well as the nutritional and medicinal values of a great many plants. It covers well-known plants and obscure varieties.)

Source, Anita Holmes. *Plant Life: 10 Easy Plants to Grow Indoors.* New York: Four Winds Press, 1974.

Sunset Magazine. San Mateo, Calif.: Lane Publishers, ongoing series. This publisher produces many books on plants and gardening, which are widely available at nurseries, in bookstores, and at the library.

10

Some Final Thoughts

This book is intended to assist all concerned individuals in their efforts to improve the quality of care and the quality of life for an increasing number of older adults in the community who need to be provided with basic services if they are to escape early or inappropriate placement in a skilled nursing facility. To be sure, homes that specialize in skilled nursing care have a vital role to play in modern health-care delivery—we couldn't image what society would be like without them—as our elderly population continues to live longer in spite of disabilities (e.g., illnesses, injuries, and the like) that, years ago, would have been fatal. But before sophisticated levels of skilled nursing care are needed, board and cares and similar residential care facilities can fill a significant gap in health care by providing the elderly with safe, comfortable, and affordable living arrangements. We hope that every community will join our efforts to help board and care managers/operators create a stimulating environment in which residents, staff, families, and the community at large can interact and grow.

Yet it must be remembered that many board and care residents remain housed in the facility with little or no encouragement to use their sensory faculties, to exercise their minds and bodies, or to accept the challenge of getting the most out of life. On the contrary, many have actually been discouraged in this regard: remarks by overworked caregivers, frustrated family members, and others with whom they come in contact leave older adults feeling as though an improved quality of life is beyond their grasp. This state of affairs is not only lamentable, it is intolerable; its destructive effects must be stopped.

Society stands frustrated, confused, and outraged at the plight of its elderly, yet we, its members, perpetrate its most heinous indignities: we degrade and demoralize, devalue and disregard; often we throw human beings on the social scrapheap with less thought than it takes to dispose of unwanted wrapping paper after the holidays. In part this is due to our deepseated fear of growing old. Aging inevitably leads to the unthinkable, death. If we can just forestall age, death will remain at bay. Oh, how childlike we are to think that by clutching at youth we can somehow deny the march of time. Deriding age will not make it go away. Acting as though it doesn't exist will not alter the truth of our own mortality.

Is it any wonder, then, that so many older people in our society are fearful, confused, and devoid of any semblance of self-esteem? The elderly are often suspicious of those who step forward to offer help. It is to be expected that board and care residents will be somewhat reluctant to embrace activities. But there is no need to be discouraged. Progress must be measured by the inch, or fraction of an inch, rather than in leaps and bounds.

We must change our ideas about the meaning of success. When a courageous individual overcomes paralysis to raise a cup and take a sip of liquid unassisted—that's success! Being unsure and cautious, if not downright suspicious (and who can blame them?), the elderly rely on psychological barriers to protect themselves from the risks involved in embarking upon new experiences. But if approached with patience, kindness, thoughtfulness, encouragement, love, and sincerity, these elders will see that there is nothing to fear from those who truly care about their needs and have a compelling desire to help.

There is much that you, the reader, can do to improve and expand the role of board and cares in your area:

- Be an advocate for the improvement of existing residential care facilities in your vicinity. Given the housing and care needs of America's elderly population, the role of board and cares will significantly increase in years to come.

- Become knowledgeable about board and cares. Read more about this growing alternative to traditional housing and care options.

- Share your time and talent to help change the quality of life for board and care residents who live near you. Maybe you could help lead an activity. Volunteers are vital: they augment the small staffs of these facilities and add so much to the lives of residents.

- Become knowledgeable about legislation in your state to bring about positive changes in existing residential care facilities, whether it be stiffer penalties for elder abuse, assuring adequate reimbursement for owners/operators, training programs for staff members, mandating improved standards for the physical structure of the home, or increased safety requirements inside the facility. Support positive legislation to make board and cares better places for all residents.

- Do what you can to help monitor the care and services of existing board and cares, not only by praising those facilities whose owners/operators are doing a good job to enhance the well-being of their residents, but also by bringing pressure to bear on less adequate homes by alerting the public to the unacceptable conditions, offering to work with the home to improve housing and/or levels of care, or, if need be, lodging a complaint with the local long-term care ombudsman.

- If you plan to choose the board and care living arrangement for yourself or a loved one, be a good consumer and shop wisely. Visit several facilities and be aware of what to look for (see Appendices 1 and 2).

The need for alternative housing to meet the demand of America's growing elderly population is not only continuous but increasing, and is supported by demographic projections. The segment of our older population classified as the "frail elderly" will double in the next thirty years, reaching seven million by the year 2030. Many older people do not need the intensive care provided by skilled nursing facilities, yet they are unable to afford many of the medium- to high-priced retirement options. For the majority of elder Americans who rely solely on Social Security for income, the less costly yet supportive living arrangement that board and cares provide may be the best available alternative to the uncertainty of living alone and the far more drastic step of nursing home placement.

After reaching the decision that a board and care is the right choice for you or your loved one, maintaining a good quality of care in the residential facility will require that physical safety, good nutrition, and proper medical attention be augmented with a well-developed program of activity to maintain the very highest level of individual well-being. It is our hope that this volume has assisted in both of these vital endeavors.

RESOURCES

Birrew, J. *The Psychology of Aging*. Englewood Cliffs, N.J.: Prentice-Hall, 1964.

Brown, P. D. and D. L. Seigal. *Ourselves, Growing Older*. Midlife and Older Women Project, New York: Simon and Schuster, 1987.

Dobkin, L. *The Board and Care System: A Regulatory Jungle*. Washington, D.C.: American Association of Retired Persons, 1989.

Gaberlavage, G., M. Moon, and S. J. Newman, eds. *Preserving Independence, Supporting Needs: The Role of Board and Care Homes*. Washington, D.C.: American Association of Retired Persons, 1988.

Galton, L. *Don't Give Up on an Aging Parent*. New York: Crown Publishers, 1975.

Haske, Margaret. *A Home Away from Home: Consumer Information on Board and Care Homes*. Washington, D.C.: American Association of Retired Persons, 1986.

Newcomer, R. and R. Stone. "Board and Care Housing: Expansion and Improvement Needed." *Generations* (Summer 1985):38–39.

Reichstein, K. J. and L. Bergosky. "Domiciliary Care Facilities for Adults: An Analysis of State and Regulations." *Research on Aging* vol. 5.

Appendix 1

What You Need to Know about Retirement Facilities

Ruby MacDonald

Whether you're looking at retirement living for yourself or your parent, here are some pertinent questions to ask and observations to make while you're touring retirement facilities so you'll pick the right one.

1. When you drive up to the facility, what is your first impression? Do you see people outdoors dozing on benches or chairs? What is the neighborhood like? Is it safe to take walks outdoors? Is the outdoor furniture chained down to prevent theft? How old is the facility? Would you be proud to live in this kind of environment?

2. When you enter the lobby, do you see people sleeping in chairs? Are there wheelchairs and walkers? Are the residents full of vitality and enthusiasm or lifeless? Would you or your parent fit into that environment? What is the overall feeling you get from the inside of the building—furniture, management, and residents? Is the furniture cheerful? Is it sturdy?

3. What is the management staff like when you walk up to the front desk? [Are they] warm, friendly, genuine? Do they have good rapport with the

From *Senior Spectrum* (August 1988):18. Reprinted by permission of the author and the publisher.

Ruby MacDonald is the author of "Power Programs," a small group support system and study program based on *The Power of Positive Thinking* by Norman Vincent Peale. The program is designed to help seniors help themselves. For information write to: Power Programs, 597 Center Avenue #100, Martinez, CA 94553.

residents? Do the residents seem to like the management team? Do the residents look happy?

4. Does the tour director appear overly anxious to rent you an apartment? Are all of your questions answered directly? Does the tour director have an in-depth understanding of what a retirement facility is all about? Has management asked what [your] real need [is] or [that of] your parent?

5. Ask if you can have a complimenary lunch or dinner to sample the food. Do they serve low-salt, low-fat, low-cholesterol meals? [What about] dietetic meals? [Are the meals served] restaurant style or cafeteria style? How many choices of entrees [are there] per meal? Check out the kitchen—is it clean and orderly? How important is good nutrition here? Is [the] dining room open or assigned seating? Are beverages available all day?

6. What is the policy about having guests in the dining room? Is there a charge? How often can you have guests and with how much notice? Is there a private dining room for family get-togethers? What are the charges [for using this room]? Are smoking and drinking [alcoholic beverages] allowed? Is there a social hour? [If so,] how often?

7. Is there a residents' council? How much voice do residents have? What are the committees? Is there a welcoming committee? Is there a residents' suggestion box?

8. [If the facility produces one,] ask for and study the monthly newsletter. How many programs are offered? What kind of outside activities are offered and how often? Is there scheduled transportation? [Are there] overnight trips? [Are there] day trips? [Are there] no-host vacation trips?

9. Does the newsletter list birthdays of residents as well as [the] names of new residents?

10. After your tour, linger and talk to the residents in the living room, or to those walking about. Ask questions. What kind of feeling do you get from them? Are they happy living there?

11. Are residents stagnating or being challenged through various intellectual, physical, spiritual, or menta [ly challenging] programs? Would these programs interest you or your parent?

12. Is everything clean and well kept, both inside and out[side of the facility]?

13. About money: is your deposit refundable? How long will your deposit hold the unit of your choice? When will rents increase? Is this a monthly rental agreement or a lease? How much notice is required if you decide to move out? Will that [moving out] cost you anything? Is there a yearly cleaning fee? Must you make a down payment [on any fees]? Is this a buy-in [much like a condominium]? If it's a buy-in, what do you get for your money that you wouldn't get on a month-to-month rental [basis]? (Most senior adults need their capital to live on rather than [to] invest in housing.)

14. Is there a room for overnight guests? What is the policy and charge?

15. How secure is the building? Are the main doors locked after dark? Do residents have a key to unlock outside doors to easily reenter the building at night?

16. How are emergencies handled? Is there an emergency alarm system in each room? How long does it take the on-duty person to respond to an emergency? Is there someone on duty twenty-four hours? Is there someone on duty and awake at all times, or a resident manager who sleeps at night? Does the staff administer CPR [cardiopulmonary resuscitation]? How long does it take for an ambulance [or the] fire department to respond to emergencies?

17. Should you need a temporary wheelchair or walker, what is the policy? Does this facility have residential-care units if more care is eventually needed?

18. Who pays for cable TV or telephone services and other utilities [the facility or the resident]?

19. Are parking facilities ample for your car and [for those of your] guests?

It is a good idea to make a written list of your expectations and needs. Then check [them] against the services actually provided before you decide on a specific retirement facility.

It pays off for everyone if you do your homework beforehand. A retirement center is good only if it's a benefit to you and your family. Always focus on these benefits while you tour various facilities.

Having been associated for many years with facilities that provide varying levels and degrees of eldercare, we heartily endorse Ms. MacDonald's suggested questions and concerns. Though it may at first seem like you are going to a lot of trouble to investigate these issues, if you keep in mind that this may well be the last home you or your loved one will ever live in, the time and effort expended to find the right facility could spell the difference between a future filled with happiness and years of boredom and frustration. Gaining the clearest possible picture of which services are available and which are not can help avoid disappointment after moving in.

We cannot stress enough that the elderly and/or their families should embark upon their search for suitable alternative housing and care long before circumstances force a quick and often ill-advised choice. The decision to relocate is never an easy one to make, and the stress is too often aggravated by the fact that care needs must be given priority. For this very reason all of us should increase our options by planning ahead. Try to be as realistic as you can about your income: housing is one of the largest portions of anyone's expenses, so you need to stay within your means.

Appendix 2

A Checklist to Take with You
When You Visit a Residential Care Facility

Dorothy Epstein

GENERAL ATMOSPHERE

_____ Do facility administration and staff respond to the presence of the Ombudsman Program positively?

_____ Are visitors welcome, in general?

_____ Are residents allowed to move freely within the facility?

_____ Do residents interact with one another? With visitors?

_____ Is [the] general atmosphere warm and hospitable?

_____ Is television on continuously?

_____ Do residents seem withdrawn and bored, or interested and involved in their lives?

_____ Is there an effort to make the facility comfortable and homelike?

_____ Is there a noticeable attitude of caring expressed toward residents by [the] manager or owner?

This checklist was written and compiled by Dorothy Epstein, Ombudsman, Inc., and is reprinted from "When Help Is Needed," a publication of the Alameda County Ombudsman, with support from the State Ombudsman and the Department on Aging, and made possible by a grant from the Junior League of Oakland/East Bay, Inc., 1989.

_____ Is [the] owner or manager readily available to discuss and resolve concerns/problems/complaints, with [the] Ombudsman?

PHYSICAL PLANT

_____ Is [the] facility clean and free of odor?

_____ Is [the] facility maintained at a comfortable temperature for residents?

_____ Is [the] facility reasonably uncluttered?

_____ Is [the] furniture clean and in good repair?

QUALITY OF CARE

_____ Does [the] physical condition of residents reflect good hygiene and adequate basic care?

_____ Are residents dressed in street clothes which appear presentable?

_____ Are residents able to get physical exercise?

RESIDENTS' RIGHTS

_____ Is privacy assured when residents receive guests?

_____ Are residents treated with dignity and respect?

_____ Can residents make and receive *private* phone calls?

_____ Do residents seem free to raise concerns or complaints without fear of retaliation?

_____ Do residents appear to have been "coached" about what to say to an Qmbudsman?

_____ Does [the] owner/manager respect resident privacy by knocking before entering a resident's bedroom?

DIETARY

_____ Are meals appetizing?

_____ Is [the] quantity sufficient?

_____ Is there variety in the menu?

_____ Are fresh fruits and vegetables used in season?

_____ Are between-meal snacks made available?

_____ Do residents dine together (as opposed to eating alone in [their] rooms)?

_____ Are residents' food preferences and cultural or religious backgrounds taken into consideration in meal planning?

ACTIVITIES

_____ Does [the] facility have a planned activity program for residents?

_____ Do meaningful social, leisure-time, physical, and educational activities take place?

MISCELLEANEOUS

_____ Is the Ombudsman poster displayed where residents and visitors can easily read it?

_____ How is personal spending money made available to residents ($66/month for SSI recipients*)?

---

*This amount may change depending on one's state of residence.

Appendix 3

State Units on Aging

Each state has its own agency that deals primarily or exclusively with matters pertaining to older persons. These agency headquarters can be contacted to secure additional information about services in your immediate vicinity, and community resources available to assist the elderly. *This list was compiled from material submitted by Ms. Cathy Schiman, Program Associate for The National Center for State Long Term Care Ombudsman Resources (Washington, D.C.). The authors are grateful for the Center's cooperation in providing this data.*

ALABAMA

Commission on Aging
Second Floor
136 Catoma Street
Montgomery, AL 36130
(205) 242-5743

ALASKA

Older Alaskans Commission
Department of Administration
Pouch C-Mail Station 0209
Juneau, AK 99811-0209
(907) 465-3250

ARIZONA

Aging and Adult Administration
Department of Economic Security
1400 West Washington Street
Phoenix, AZ 85007
(602) 542-4446

ARKANSAS

Division of Aging and Adult Services
Arkansas Department of Human
    Services
P.O. Box 1417, SLOT 1412
7th and Main Streets
Little Rock, AR 72201
(501) 682-2441

CALIFORNIA

Department of Aging
1600 K Street
Sacramento, CA 95814
(916) 322-5290

COLORADO

Aging and Adult Services
Department of Social Services
1575 Sherman Street, 10th Floor
Denver, CO 80203-1714
(303) 866-3851

CONNECTICUT

Commissioner
Department of Aging
175 Main Street
Hartford, CT 06106
(203) 566-3238

DELAWARE

Division on Aging
Department of Health and Social
    Services
1901 North DuPont Highway
New Castle, DE 19720
(302) 421-6791

DISTRICT OF COLUMBIA

Office on Aging
1424 K. Street N.W.
2nd Floor
Washington, D.C. 20005
(202) 724-5626

FLORIDA

Program Office of Aging and Adult
    Services
Department of Health and Rehabilita-
    tive Services
1317 Winewood Boulevard
Tallahassee, FL 32301
(904) 488-8922

GEORGIA

Office of Aging
878 Peachtree Street, N.E.
Rm. 632
Atlanta, GA 30309
(404) 894-5333

HAWAII

Executive Office on Aging
Office of the Governor
335 Merchant Street, Rm. 241
Honolulu, HI 96813
(808) 548-2593

IDAHO

Office on Aging
Rm. 108—Statehouse
Boise, ID 83720
(208) 334-3833

ILLINOIS

Department on Aging
421 East Capitol Avenue
Springfield, IL 62701
(217) 785-2870

INDIANA

Division of Aging Services
Department of Human Services
251 North Illinois Street
P.O. Box 7083
Indianapolis, IN 46207-7083
(317) 232-7020

IOWA

Department of Elder Affairs
Suite 236, Jewett Building
914 Grand Avenue
Des Moines, IA 50319
(515) 281-5187

KANSAS

Department on Aging
Docking State Office Building, 122-S
915 S.W. Harrison
Topeka, KS 66612-1500
(913) 296-4986

KENTUCKY

Division of Aging Services
Cabinet for Human Resources
CHR Building—6th West
275 East Main Street
Frankfort, KY 40621
(502) 564-6930

LOUISIANA

Office of Elderly Affairs
4550 N. Boulevard, 2nd Floor
P.O. Box 80374
Baton Rouge, LA 70806
(504) 925-1700

MAINE

Director
Bureau of Elder & Adult Services
Department of Human Services
State House—Station #11
Augusta, ME 04333
(207) 626-5335

MARYLAND

Office on Aging
State Office Building
301 West Preston Street, Rm. 1004
Baltimore, MD 21201
(301) 225-1100

MASSACHUSETTS

Executive Office of Elder Affairs
38 Chauncy Street
Boston, MA 02111
(617) 727-7750

MICHIGAN

Office of Services to the Aging
P.O. Box 30026
Lansing, MI 48909
(517) 373-8230

MINNESOTA

Board on Aging
444 Lafayette Road
St. Paul, MN 55155-3843
(612) 296-2770

MISSISSIPPI

Council on Aging
Division of Aging and Adult Services
421 West Pascagoula Street
Jackson, MS 39203-3524
(601) 949-2070

MISSOURI

Division on Aging
Department of Social Services
P.O. Box 1337
2701 West Main Street
Jefferson City, MO 65102
(314) 751-3082

MONTANA

The Governor's Office on Aging
State Capitol Building
Capitol Station, Room 219
Helena, MT 59620
(406) 444-3111

NEBRASKA

Department on Aging
P.O. Box 95044
301 Centennial Mall-South
Lincoln, NE 68509
(402) 471-2306

NEVADA

Division for Aging Services
Department of Human Resources
340 North 11th Street, Suite 114
Las Vegas, NV 89101
(702) 486-3545

NEW HAMPSHIRE

Division of Elderly & Adult Services
6 Hazen Drive
Concord, NH 03301-6501
(603) 271-4680

NEW JERSEY

Division on Aging
Department of Community Affairs
CN807
South Broad and Front Streets
Trenton, NJ 08625-0807
(609) 292-4833

NEW MEXICO

State Agency on Aging
224 East Palace Avenue, 4th Floor
La Villa Rivera Building
Santa Fe, NM 87501
(505) 827-7640

NEW YORK

Office for the Aging
New York State Plaza
Agency Building #2
Albany, NY 12223
(518) 474-4425

NORTH CAROLINA

Division of Aging
693 Palmer Drive
Raleigh, NC 27603
(919) 733-3983

NORTH DAKOTA

Aging Services
Department of Human Services
State Capitol Building
Bismarck, ND 58505
(701) 224-2577

OHIO

Department of Aging
50 West Broad Street, 9th Floor
Columbus, OH 43266-0501
(614) 466-5500

OKLAHOMA

Aging Services Division
Department of Human Services
P.O. Box 25352
Oklahoma City, OK 73125
(405) 521-2327

OREGON

Senior and Disabled Services Division
313 Public Service Building
Salem, OR 97310
(503) 378-4728

PENNSYLVANIA

Department of Aging
231 State Street
Harrisburg, PA 17101-1195
(717) 783-1550

PUERTO RICO

Governor's Office for Elderly Affairs
Call Box 50063
Old San Juan Station
San Juan, PR 00902
(809) 721-5710

RHODE ISLAND

Department of Elderly Affairs
160 Pine Street
Providence, RI 02903-3708
(401) 277-2858

SOUTH CAROLINA

Commission on Aging
Suite B-500
400 Arbor Lake Drive
Columbia, SC 29223
(803) 735-0210

SOUTH DAKOTA

Office of Adult Services and Aging
700 North Illinois Street
Kneip Building
Pierre, SD 57501
(605) 773-3656

TENNESSEE

Commission on Aging
Suite 201
706 Church Street
Nashville, TN 37243-0860
(615) 741-2056

TEXAS

Department on Aging
P.O. Box 12786 Capitol Station
1949 IH 35, South
Austin, TX 78741-3702
(512) 444-2727

UTAH

Division of Aging and Adult Services
Department of Social Services
120 North–200 West
Box 45500
Salt Lake City, UT 84145-0500
(801) 538-3910

VERMONT

Department of Rehabilitation & Aging
103 South Main Street
Waterbury, VT 05676
(802) 241-2400

VIRGINIA

Department for the Aging
700 Centre, 10th Floor
700 East Franklin Street
Richmond, VA 23219-2327
(804) 225-2271

WASHINGTON

Aging and Adult Services
    Administration
Department of Social and Health
    Services
OB-44A
Olympia, WA 98504
(206) 586-3768

WEST VIRGINIA

Commission on Aging
Holly Grove-State Capitol
Charleston, WV 25305
(304) 348-3317

WISCONSIN

Bureau of Aging
Division of Community Services
217 South Hamilton Street
Suite 300
Madison, WI 53707
(608) 266-2536

WYOMING

Commission on Aging
Hathaway Building, Rm. 139
Cheyenne, WY 82002-0710
(307) 777-7986

Appendix 4

State Agencies with Jurisdiction over Residential Care Facilities

The following is a list of state agencies whose jurisdictions include residential care facilities. These offices can also be valuable sources for board and care residents and their families. *This list is adapted from materials supplied by The National Association of Residential Care Facilities. The authors wish to thank NARCF President Winona Hardy for her valuable assistance.*

ALABAMA

Department of Public Health
Division of Licensure and Certification
Rm. 654 State Office Bldg.
501 Dexter Avenue
Montgomery, AL 36130
(205) 261-5113

State Department of Human
    Resources
Adult Services Division
64 North Union Street
Montgomery, Al 36130

ALASKA

Division of Family & Youth Services
Department of Health & Social
    Services
Rm. 222, MacKay Bldg.
338 Denali
Anchorage, AK 99501
(907) 274-5686

ARIZONA

Bureau of Health Care Institute
    License
Department of Health Services
Birch Hall
411 N. 24th Street
Phoenix, AZ 85008
(602) 255-4791

Department of Economic Security
Division of Development Disabilities
1400 W. Washington Street
P.O. Box 6760
Phoenix, AZ 85005
(602) 255-4791

ARKANSAS

Department of Developmental
Disabilities Services
Suite 400, Walden Bldg.
Little Rock, AR 72201
(501) 371-3416

Department of Human Services
Division of Economic & Medical Long
    Term Care
P.O. Box 1437
Donaghey Bldg., Ste. 421
Little Rock, AR 72203
(501) 371-8143

CALIFORNIA

Department of Social Services
Community Care Licensure
1315 5th Street, 5th Floor
Sacramento, CA 95814
(916) 324-4053

COLORADO

Colorado Department of Social
    Services
Aging & Adult Services Division
P.O. Box 181000
Denver, CO 80218-0899
(303) 294-5905

Department of Health
Health Facility Regulation
4210 E. 11th Avenue, Rm. 352
Denver, CO 80220
(303) 320-8333

CONNECTICUT

Department of Health Services
Hospital & Medical Care Division
150 Washington Street
Hartford, CT 06106
(203) 566-5969

DELAWARE

Department of Health & Social
    Services
1901 N. Dupont Highway
New Castle, DE 19808
(302) 421-6101

Bureau of Health Facility License
Division of Public Health
1901 N. Dupont Highway
New Castle, DE 19808
(302) 995-6674

DISTRICT OF COLUMBIA

Department of Human Services
Service Facility Regulation
    Administration
614 H. Street, N.W. Rm. 1014
Washington, DC 20001
(202) 727-7236

Department of Human Services
Long Term Care Administration
Infirmary One South
No. 2, D.C. Village Lane, S.W.
Washington, DC 20032
(202) 767-8356

FLORIDA

Office of Licensure & Certification
2727 Mahan Drive
Tallahassee, FL 32308
(904) 487-1004
(904) 488-2650

Department of Aging & Adult Services
1317 Winewood Blvd.
Tallahassee, FL 32301
(904) 488-3673

GEORGIA

Long-Term Care Ombudsman
Office of Aging
878 Peachtree Street, N.E.
Rm. 642
Atlanta, GA 30309
(404) 894-5336

Department of Human Resources
ORS Compliance Monitoring,
878 Peachtree Street, N.E.
Suite 810
Atlanta, GA 30309
(404) 894-4775

HAWAII

Department of Social Services &
   Housing
P.O. Box 339
Honolulu, HI 96809
(808) 548-5902

Hospital, Medical Facilities Branch
Department of Health
P.O. Box 3378
1250 Punchbowl Street
Honolulu, HI 96801
(808) 548-5902

IDAHO

Facility Standards Program
Department of Health & Welfare
420 W. Washington
Boise, ID 83720
(208) 334-4169

ILLINOIS

Long Term Care Section
Department of Public Health
525 W. Jefferson
Springfield, IL 62761
(217) 782-5180

INDIANA

State Board of Health
Division of Health Facilities
1330 W. Michigan Street
Indianapolis, IN 46204
(317) 633-8442

IOWA

Licensing & Certification
Department of Health
Lucas St. Office Bldg.
Des Moines, IA 50319
(515) 281-4129

Department of Inspections & Appeals
Lucas St. Office Bldg., 2nd Floor
Des Moines, IA 50319
(515) 281-4129

Health Facilities Division
Lucas St. Office Bldg., 2nd Floor
Des Moines, IA 50319
(515) 281-4115

KANSAS

Department of Health & Environment
Landon State Office Bldg.
900 S.W. Jackson, 10th Floor
Topeka, KS 66620
(913) 862-9360

KENTUCKY

Division of Licensing & Regulations
Department of Human Resources
275 E. Main Street
Frankfort, KY 40621
(502) 564-2800

LOUISIANA

Governor's Office of Elderly Affairs
P.O. Box 80374
Baton Rouge, LA 70898
(504) 925-1700

MAINE

Division of Residential Care
State House Station, No. 11
Augusta, ME 04333
(207) 289-2821

Bureau of Medical Services
Department of Human Services
Augusta, ME 04333
(207) 289-2674

MARYLAND

Department of Human Resource
Office of Adult Services
300 W. Preston Street, Rm. 403
Baltimore, MD 21201
(301) 576-5276

Division of Licensing & Certification
Department of Health and Mental
    Hygiene
201 W. Preston Street
Baltimore, MD 21201
(301) 383-2517

MASSACHUSETTS

Department of Public Health
Division of Health Care Quality
11th Floor, 80 Boylston Street
Boston, MA 02116
(617) 727-5864

MICHIGAN

Bureau of Regulatory Service
Department of Social Service
P.O. Box 30037
Lansing, MI 48909
(517) 373-1400

Division of Health Facility Licensing &
    Certification
Department of Public Health
3500 N. Logan
P.O. Box 30035
Lansing, MI 48909
(517) 373-0900

MINNESOTA

Records and Information Unit
Health Systems Division
717 S.E. Delaware Street
Minneapolis, MN 55440
(612) 623-5405

Public Health Department
4176 E. Delaware Street
P.O. Box 9441
Minneapolis, MN 55440
(612) 296-5442

Division of Licensing
Department of Human Services
444 Lafayette Rd.
Space Center Bldg.
St. Paul, MN 55101
(612) 297-3000

MISSISSIPPI

Health Care Commission
Mississippi Department of Health
Division of Health Facilities Licensure
P.O. Box 1700
Jackson, MS 39205
(601) 960-7769

MISSOURI

Missouri Division of Aging
Licensure Unit
505 Missouri Blvd.
Jefferson City, MO 65101
(314) 751-4480

MONTANA

Food & Consumer Safety Bureau
Department of Health & Environmental Services
Cogswell Bldg.
Helena, MT 56920
(406) 449-2408

Health Services Division
Department of Health & Environmental Services
Cogswell Bldg.
Helena, MT 56920
(406) 499-2037

Department of Family Services
48 N. Last Chance Gulch
P.O. Box 8005
Helena, MT 59604
(406) 444-5900

NEBRASKA

Aged & Disabled Services
P.O. Box 95026
Lincoln, NE 68509
(402) 471-3121

Division of Licensure & Standards
Department of Health
Box 95007
801 Centennial Mall S.
Lincoln, NE 68509
(402) 471-2946

NEVADA

State Welfare Division
251 Jeanell
Capitol Complex
Carson City, NV 89710
(702) 885-4184

Bureau of Regulatory Health Services
Department of Human Resources
505 East King Street, Rm. 202
Carson City, NV 89710
(702) 885-4474

NEW HAMPSHIRE

Division of Public Health
Bureau of Health Facilities
6 Hazen Drive
Concord, NH 03301
(603) 271-4592

NEW JERSEY

Department of Community Affairs
Bureau of Room & Board House
    Standards
363 W. State Street, CN 804
Trenton, NJ 08625
(609) 987-4262

State Department of Health
Licensing & Certification
CN 367
Trenton, NJ 08625
(609) 292-4304

NEW MEXICO

Licensing Health Related Facilities
P.O. Box 968
Kennedy Hall
Santa Fe, NM 87503
(505) 827-3431

NEW YORK

Department of Social Services
Bureau of Residential Services
44 Holland Avenue
Albany, NY 12229
(518) 473-4100

Department of Social Services
Division of Adult Services
Fl. 9A, 40 North Pearl Street
Albany, NY 12243
(518) 474-9468

NORTH CAROLINA

Department of Human Resources
Division of Facility Services
701 Barbour Drive
Raleigh, NC 27603
(919) 733-4660

NORTH DAKOTA

Department of Human Services
State Capital Bldg.
Bismarck, ND 58505
(701) 224-2321

Department of Human Services
Aging Services
State Capital Bldg.
Bismarck, ND 58505
(701) 224-2577

OHIO

Division of Department of Health
Licensing & Certification
P.O. Box 118
246 N. High Street
Columbus, OH 43266-0118
(614) 466-2070

Bureau of Licensing & Standards
Department of Human Services
30 E. Broad Street
Columbus, OH 43215
(614) 466-8748

OKLAHOMA

Room & Board Home License
    Division
Department of Health
1000 N. E. 10th Street
P.O. Box 53551
Oklahoma City, OK 73152
(405) 271-6868

OREGON

Senior Services Division
313 Public Service Bldg.
Salem, OR 97310
(503) 378-3751

PENNSYLVANIA

Department of Aging
Barto Bldg.
231 State Street
Harrisburg, PA 17101
(717) 783-7999

Department of Public Welfare
Division of Standards & Quality
    Assurance
Box 2675
Harrisburg, PA 17105
(717) 783-5132

Department of Public Welfare
Personal Care Home Enforcement
    Specialist
Box 2675
Harrisburg, PA 17105
(717) 783-5132

RHODE ISLAND

Division of Facility Regulation
Rhode Island Department of Health
75 Davis Street
Providence, RI 02908
(401) 277-2566

SOUTH CAROLINA

South Carolina Department of Health
    and Environmental Control
Office of Health Licensing
2600 Bull Street
Columbia, SC 29201
(803) 734-4530

SOUTH DAKOTA

Licensing & Certification Program
Department of Health
523 E. Capital
Joe Fosse Bldg.
Pierre, SD 57501
(605) 773-3364

TENNESSEE

Board of Licensing Health Care
    Facilities
283 Plus Park Blvd.
Nashville, TN 37217
(615) 367-6316

TEXAS

Texas Department of Health
Quality Standards Division
1100 W. 49th Street
Austin, TX 78756
(512) 458-7611

UTAH

Health Facilities & Standards
150 W. North Temple
Box 2500, Suite 316
Salt Lake City, UT 84110
(801) 533-7817

Division of Aging
Department of Social Services
150 W. North Temple, Rm. 326
Salt Lake City, UT 84110
(801) 533-6422

VERMONT

Division of Licensure & Registration
103 S. Main Street
Waterbury, VT 05676
(802) 241-2158

VIRGINIA

Division of Licensing
Department of Social Services
8007 Discovery Drive
Blair Bldg.
Richmond, VA 23288
(804) 281-9025

WASHINGTON

Department of Social & Health
    Services
Bureau of Aging & Adult Services
OB430
Olympia, WA 98504
(206) 753-4921

Personal Care Facilities
Survey Section
Office of Licensing & Certification
Division of Health ET-31
DSHS
1112 South Quince Street
Olympia, WA 98504
(206) 753-5823

WEST VIRGINIA

Health Facilities Licensure
    Certification
Department of Health
1800 Washington Street, E.
Charleston, WV 25305
(304) 348-2971

Adult Services
Department of Welfare
1900 Washington Street
Charleston, WV 25305
(304) 348-7980

WISCONSIN

Department of Health & Social
    Services
Division of Community Services
Rm. 420
P.O. Box 7851
Madison, WI 53707
(608) 266-1255

WYOMING

Division of Health & Medical Services
Department of Health & Social
    Services
Hathaway Bldg., 4th Floor
Cheyenne, WY 82002
(307) 777-7121

Division of Public Assistance & Social
    Services
Hathaway Bldg.
Cheyenne, WY 82002
(307) 777-6094

Appendix 5

State Long-Term Care Ombudsman

Listed below are the names, addresses, and telephone numbers of individuals who serve as their state's Long-Term Care Ombudsman. To locate your local ombudsman, please contact the state office. *The authors wish to thank Cathy Schiman and the National Center for State Long Term Care Ombudsman Resources for providing this important information.*

ALABAMA

Patti Dake
Commission on Aging
136 Catoma Street, 2nd Floor
Montgomery, AL 36130
(205) 261-5743

ALASKA

William O'Connor
Office of the Older Alaskans
    Ombudsman
3601 C Street, Suite 260
Anchorage, AK 99508-5209
(907) 279-2232
(accepts collect calls from older
    persons)

ARIZONA

Rozz Webster
Aging and Adult Administration
P.O. Box 6123-950A
1400 West Washington Street
Phoenix, AZ 85007
(602) 542-4446

ARKANSAS

Raymon Harvey
Division of Aging and Adult Services
1417 Donaghey Plaza South—
    POB 1437
7th and Maine Streets
Little Rock, AR 72203-1437
(501) 682-8952

CALIFORNIA

Sterling Boyer
California Department on Aging
1600 K Street
Sacramento, CA 95814
(916) 323-6681
(800) 231-4024

COLORADO

Virginia Fraser
The Legal Center
455 Sherman Street, Suite 130
Denver, CO 80203
(303) 722-0300
(800) 332-6356

CONNECTICUT

Ida Arbitman
Connecticut Department on Aging
175 Main Street
Hartford, CT 06106
(203) 566-7770

DELAWARE

Marietta Z. Wooleyhan
Division on Aging
1113 Church Avenue
Milford, DE 19963
(302) 422-1386
(800) 223-9074

DISTRICT OF COLUMBIA

Bruce Vignery
Legal Counsel for the Elderly
1909 K Street, N.W.
Washington, DC 20049
(202) 662-4933

FLORIDA

Barbara Pogge
State LTC Ombudsman Council
Office of the Governor
154 Holland Building
Tallahassee, FL 32399-0001
(904) 488-6190

GEORGIA

Joanne Mathis
Office of Aging
Department of Human Resources
878 Peachtree Street, N.W., Rm. 632
Atlanta, GA 30389
(404) 894-5336

HAWAII

Sandy Rongitsch
Hawaii Executive Office on Aging
335 Merchant Street, Rm. 241
Honolulu, HI 96813
(808) 548-2539

IDAHO

Arlene Davidson
Office on Aging
State House, Rm. 114
Boise, ID 83720
(208) 334-3833

IOWA

Carl McPherson
Department of Elder Affairs
Jewett Building, Suite 236
916 Grand Avenue
Des Moines, IA 50319
(515) 281-5187

ILLINOIS

Neyna Johnson
Department on Aging
421 East Capitol Avenue
Springfield, IL 62701
(217) 785-3140

INDIANA

Robin Grant
Division of Aging
Department of Human Services
251 N. Illinois—POB 7083
Indianapolis, IN 46207-7083
(317) 232-7020
(800) 622-4484

KANSAS

Myron Dunavan
Department on Aging
Docking State Office Building, 122-S
915 S.W. Harrison
Topeka, KS 66612-1500
(913) 296-4986
(800) 432-3535

KENTUCKY

Gary Hammonds
Division for Aging Services
Cabinet for Human Resources
CHR Building—6th Ploor, West
275 East Main Street
Frankfort, KY 40621
(502) 564-6930
(800) 372-2291

LOUISIANA

Hugh Eley
Governor's Office of Elderly Affairs
4528 Bennington Avenue, Box 80374
Baton Rouge, LA 70898-3074
(504) 925-1700

MAINE

Joan Sturmthal
Maine Commission on Aging
State House, Station 127
Augusta, ME 04333
(207) 289-3658
(800) 452-1912

MARYLAND

Condict Stevenson
Office on Aging
301 West Preston Street, Rm. 1
Baltimore, MD 21201
(301) 225-1083

MASSACHUSETTS

Susan McDonough
Executive Office of Elder Affairs
38 Chauncy Street
Boston, MA 02111
(617) 727-7273

MICHIGAN

Hollis Turnham
Citizens for Better Care
1627 East Kalamazoo
Lansing, MI 48912
(517) 482-1297
(800) 292-7852

MINNESOTA

Jim Varpness
Board on Aging
Office of Ombudsman for Older
    Minnesotans
444 Lafayette Road
St. Paul, MN 55155-3843
(612) 296-7465
(800) 652-9747

MISSISSIPPI

Cinda Martin
Council on Aging
421 West Pascagoula
Jackson, MS 39203
(601) 949-2070

MISSOURI

Carol Scott
Division of Aging
Department of Social Services
P.O. Box 1337
2701 W. Main Street
Jefferson City, MO 65102
(314) 751-3082

MONTANA

Doug Blakley
Seniors' Office of Legal and Ombuds-
    man Services
P.O. Box 232, Capitol Station
Helena, MT 59620
(406) 444-4676
(800) 332-2272

NEBRASKA

Geri Tucker
Department on Aging
P.O. Box 95044
301 Centennial Mall South
Lincoln, NE 68509-5044
(402) 471-2306
(402) 471-2307

NEVADA

Earl Yamashita
Division of Aging Services
Department of Human Resources
Kinkead Building, Rm. 101
Carson City, NV 89710
(702) 885-4210

NEW HAMPSHIRE

Gyme Hardy
Division of Elderly and Adult Services
6 Hazen Drive
Concord, NH 03301-6508
(603) 271-4375
(800) 442-5640

NEW JERSEY

Harold George
Office of the Ombudsman for the Insti-
    tutionalized Elderly
28 West State Street, Rm. 305
CN808
Trenton, NJ 08625-0807
(609) 292-8016
(800) 624-4262

NEW MEXICO

Janet Rose
State Agency on Aging
LaVilla Rivera Building, 4th Floor
224 East Palace Avenue
Santa Fe, NM 87501
(505) 827-7640

NEW YORK

Dave Murray
Office for the Aging
Agency Building, #2
Empire State Plaza
Albany, NY 12223
(518) 474-7329

NORTH CAROLINA

Debbie Brantley
Department of Human Resources
Division of Aging
693 Palmer Drive
Raleigh, NC 27603
(919) 733-8400

NORTH DAKOTA

Jo Hildebrant
Aging Services Division
Department of Human Services
State Capitol Building
Bismarck, ND 58505
(701) 224-2577
(800) 472-2622

OHIO

Roland Hornbostel
Department of Aging
50 West Broad Street, 9th Floor
Columbus, OH 43266-0501
(614) 466-9927
(800) 282-1206

OKLAHOMA

Esther Allgood
Division of Aging Services
Department of Human Services
P.O. Box 25352
Oklahoma City, OK 73125
(405) 521-2281

OREGON

Meredith Cote
Office of LTC Ombudsman
2475 Lancaster Drive
Building B, #9
Salem, OR 97310
(503) 378-6533
(800) 522-2602

PENNSYLVANIA

Linda Jackman
Department of Aging
Barto Building
231 State Street
Harrisburg, PA 17101
(717) 783-7247

PUERTO RICO

Norma Venegas
Governor's Office on Elderly Affairs
Call Box 50063
Old San Juan Station, PR 00902
(809) 722-2429

RHODE ISLAND

Catherine Callahan
Department of Elderly Affairs
160 Pine Street
Providence, RI 02903-3708
(401) 277-6883

SOUTH CAROLINA

Mary B. Fagan
Office of the Governor
Division of Ombudsman and Citizens'
    Service
1205 Pendleton Street
Columbia, SC 29201
(803) 734-0457

SOUTH DAKOTA

Rolland Hostler
Office of Adult Services and Aging
Department of Social Services
Richard F. Kneip Building
700 North Illinois Street
Pierre, SD 57501-2291
(605) 773-3656

TENNESSEE

Jane Bridgman
Commission on Aging
706 Church Street, Suite 201
Nashville, TN 37219-5573
(615) 741-2056

TEXAS

John Willis
Department on Aging
P.O. Box 12786 Capitol Station
1949 IH 35, South
Austin, TX 78741-3702
(512) 444-2727
(800) 252-9240

UTAH

Marj Drury
Division of Aging & Adult Services
Department of Social Services
120 North—200 West, Box 45500
Salt Lake City, UT 84145-0500
(801) 538-3920

VERMONT

Camille George
Office on Aging
108 South Main Street
Waterbury, VT 05676
(802) 241-2400
(800) 642-5119

VIRGINIA

Virginia Dize
Department for the Aging
10th Floor
700 East Franklin Street
Richmond, VA 23219-2327
(804) 225-2271
(800) 552-3402

WASHINGTON

Kary Hyre
South King County
Multi-Service Center
1200 South, 336 Street
Federal Way, WA 98003
(206) 838-6810
(800) 422-1384

WEST VIRGINIA

Carolyn Riffle
Commission on Aging
State Capitol Complex
Charleston, WV 25805
(304) 348-3317

WISCONSIN

George Potaracke
Board on Aging and Long Term Care
214 North Hamilton Street
Madison, WI 53703
(608) 266-8944

WYOMING

Debra Alden
Wyoming State Bar Association
900 8th Street
Wheatland, WY 82201
(307) 322-5553

Appendix 6

A Sample Order of Worship

A word of thanks:

God, our Creator, we thank you for this opportunity to come together to share our concerns for one another and to join in praise and thanksgiving for your many gifts to us.

AMEN

A hymn of praise:

Possibly "All People that on Earth Do Dwell" or some other appropriate selection.

Collective prayer followed by the Lord's Prayer:

At this time ask if anyone has a concern or specific joy to share, someone for whom they want a special prayer, or expressions of specific needs.

O God, who hears all the pains in our hearts, bring comfort to us. You who know our deepest joys, be with us so that we may share our joys with our sisters and brothers.

_____ has had to go to the hospital for surgery. Bring healing to his/her body. Comfort the family that they may be a source of strength to him/her.

_____ has a new great-grandchild. May we all share in his/ her pride and joy and pray that this new life will grow strong and be worthy of your gifts.

_____ has lost his/her best friend. Comfort him/her in his/ her loss and pain and let _____ know that we care.

We ask these things in the name of Jesus our Lord (or substitute the phrase "in Your name") as we join our hearts and minds in love and caring for one another, in the prayer You taught us: (The Lord's Prayer is recited). (At this point in the service, a recording of the Lord's Prayer sung by any well-known performer may prove a useful change of pace.)

After the Lord's Prayer, traditionally a hymn of meditation is sung: e.g., "Just As I Am," "Spirit of God, Descend Upon My Heart," "Love Lifted Me," etc.

Today's Scripture:

Psalm 24 (or any selection from an appropriate source). (This can be the time to ask what the residents think these words mean. A discussion could take place about how this passage might apply to their lives.)

After such a discussion period, a song of dedication or closing is appropriate. Here are some suggestions:

"I Love to Tell the Story"
"Faith of Our Fathers"
"God of Love and God of Power"
"Have Thine Own Way, Lord"
"I Could Be True"
"I Am Thine, O Lord"

It can be traditional, nontraditional, modern, folk, or from some specific ethnic heritage.

Appendix 7

Songs for Music Therapy

ACTION SONGS (using hand and foot movements)

What are action songs? They are songs whose words are easily combined with various bodily motions. These movements can be as complicated as dance routines or as simple as waving one's hands and/or arms.

"This Is the Way We . . ."
(Children's learning song)

Sing and act as you remember things you do—wash your face, comb your hair, brush your teeth, reach for a bowl, etc., etc.

"We Are Climbing Jacob's Ladder"
(American Folk Hymn)

1. We are climbing Jacob's ladder. We are climbing Jacob's ladder. We are climbing Jacob's ladder, followers of the Cross.

   ["We are climbing"—use climbing motion
   "Followers of the Cross"—spread arms wide waist high. Bring left arm in front of chest, palm down flat; right hand meets left thumb at the base of the little finger, the palm of the right hand is facing left.]

2. Every round goes higher, higher. Every round goes higher, higher. Every round goes higher, higher, followers of the Cross.

   ["Every round goes"—start with hands on hips, then bring arms chest high, followed by touching fingers above the head, all the while creating a round shape.
   "Followers"—as above]

3. If you love Him, why not serve Him? If you love Him, why not serve Him? If you love Him, why not serve Him? Followers of the Cross.

["If you love Him"—arms crossed in front of chest
"Why not serve Him?—spread arms open with palms facing up and hands moving forward, as if questioning
repeat both actions twice
"Followers"—as above]

Rounds

Rounds are simple action songs that are fun to sing. The key is remembering to sing along with your group instead of a group that started a verse before or after yours. Use exaggerated, sweeping motions to act out such songs as "Three Blind Mice" or this favorite:

"Row, Row, Row Your Boat"

1. Row, row, row your boat gently down the stream;
      [Row with a circular motion in the shoulders.]
   Merrily, merrily, merrily, life is but a dream.
      [Enthusiastically throw hands up in air.]

2. Hoe, hoe, hoe your row, thru' the summer heat;
      [Use hoeing motion; wipe sweat from your brow.]
   Do your bit, cherrily stick to it, raising beans and wheat.
      [Keep hoeing; rise up as though crop is growing.]

3. Save, save, save the wheat, meat and sugar, too;
      [Throw your hands back and bring together.]
   Corn and potatoes and rice and tomatoes, are might-y good for you!
      [Pat left shoulder with right hand, right shoulder with left hand, cross arms and hug yourself.]

SPIRITUALS

Coming out of the anguish of a captive people, the spiritual expresses a yearning for safety and comfort that strikes a warm response in all of us. Based on rhythms and melodies that the African peoples brought with them, a unique form of American music came about from this mixture of cultures. The well-known campfire song "Kum Ba Yah (Come By Here)" shows this influence. And this favorite of young and old alike lends itself to low-impact movement.

"He's Got the Whole World in His Arms"

1. He's got the whole world—in His arms,
        [Spread out arms as if embracing the whole world.]
   He's got the whole world—in His arms.
   He's got the whole world—in His arms,
   He's got the whole world in His arms.

2. He's got you and me brother—in His arms,
        [Point to a man, self, then embrace.]
   He's got you and me sister—in is His arms.
        [Point to a woman, self, then embrace.]
   He's got all the children in His arms,
   He's got the whole world in His arms.

3. He's got the little bitty baby in His arms,
        [Appear to be cradling a baby in your arms.]
   He's got the little bitty baby in His arms.
   He's got the little bitty baby in His arms,
   He's got the whole world in His arms

4. He's got every-body—in His arms,
        [Sweeping motion, embrace.]
   He's got every-body—in His arms.
   He's got every-body—in His arms,
   He's got the whole world in His arms.

(Try addressing individuals in the room by name and watch their reaction. Ask if residents would like to include someone they love by name in the song.)

NONSENSE SONGS

Nonsense songs are meant to be sung for fun without having much logic or meaning. Sing them with exuberance and laughter.

"Noah's Ark"

1. Old Noah built himself an ark,
   There's one wide river to cross.
   He built it all of hick'ry bark,
   There's one wide river to cross.

Chorus

2. The animals went in one by ones
   There's one wide river to cross.
   And Japhet with a big bass drum,
   There's one wide river to cross.

Chorus

3. The animals went in two by two,
   There's one wide river to cross.
   The elephant and the kangaroo,
   There's one wide river to cross.

Chorus

4. The animals went in three by three,
   There's one wide river to cross.
   The hippopotamus and the bumble bee,
   There's one wide river to cross.

Chorus

5. And when he found they had no sail,
   There's one wide river to cross.
   He just ran up his old coat tail,
   There's one wide river to cross.

Chorus

There's one wide river, and that river is Jordan,
　　[Spread arms out wide, make flowing motion with hands.]
There's one wide river, there's one wide river to cross.
　　[Spread arms wide, make flowing motion, end with cross.]

Other fun songs include "Yankee Doodle," "My Darling Clementine," "Oh! Susanna," and "There Was a BEE-I-E-I-E."

HYMNS

Favorite hymns that express the love of God for all humans offer residents comfort and reassurance, while others are joyful and uplifting. Hymns should be a part of your sing-alongs.

"Amazing Grace"
"God Will Take Care of You"
"Just as I Am"
"Pass Me Not, O Gentle Savior"
"Balm In Gilhead"
"Love Lifted Me"

Joyous Songs

"Bringing in the Sheaves"
"Bring Them In"
"Revive Us Again"
"My Hope Is Built"

These are just a few of the many hymns that residents will enjoy singing time and time again.

Appendix 8

Friendly Visitors

These instructions are adapted from those developed by Ivy Down to assist volunteer visitors at the Salem Lutheran Home. These basic guidelines can be incorporated into any board and care environment.

DUTIES

1. Visit the assigned resident as scheduled once a week or twice a month.

2. Provide socialization activities and companionship. This may include reading to the resident, writing letters for him or her, engaging in conversation, taking walks, or enjoying the grounds.

3. Assist the resident with shopping, errands, or transportation (but only occasionally).

RESPONSIBILITIES

1. Keep a record of time spent with the resident each time you visit.

2. Wear any required name badge so you can be properly identified by the staff.

3. Observe confidentiality: if something is said to you in confidence, respect the resident's wishes.

4. Meet regularly with the volunteer coordinator.

5. If any questions or problems arise which you are not able to handle, refer them to your supervisor as soon as possible. Please do not provide advise without first consulting your supervisor.

6. Use discretion in giving the resident your home telephone number. In most cases, it is not advisable. Residents can come to the volunteer coordinator's office and leave a message.

7. Do not accept any money or gifts from residents.

8. Be relaxed. A large part of interpersonal communication is nonverbal; if you are tense, you will communicate it to the resident.

9. Listen carefully. Having someone listen to what they have to say is very important to the resident's sense of self-worth. Let the resident talk.

10. Dress comfortably and suitably. The facility is an informal place but elders are accustomed to seeing people dressed nicely, that is, clean and casual, not fancy or formal.